Ballerina Body

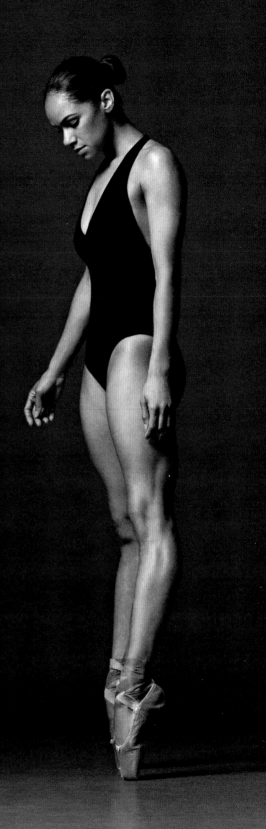

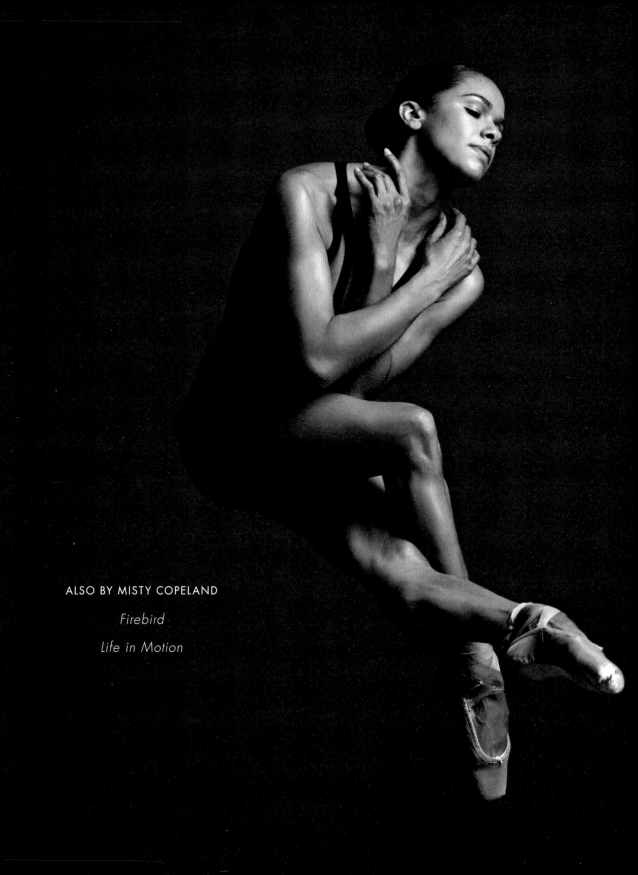

Misty Copeland

with Charisse Jones

Ballerina Body

Dancing and Eating Your Way to a
Leaner, Stronger, and More Graceful You

Movement and Dance Photography by Henry Leutwyler
Food Photography by Amy Roth

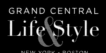

GRAND CENTRAL
Life & Style
NEW YORK · BOSTON

Copyright © 2017 by Misty Copeland
Movement and dance photographs copyright © 2017 by Henry Leutwyler
Food photographs copyright © 2017 by Amy Roth
Jacket and book design by Shubhani Sarkar, sarkardesignstudio.com
Jacket photographs copyright © Henry Leutwyler
Jacket copyright © 2017
by Hachette Book Group, Inc.

Hachette Book Group supports the right to free expression and the value of copyright. The purpose of copyright is to encourage writers and artists to produce the creative works that enrich our culture.

The scanning, uploading, and distribution of this book without permission is a theft of the author's intellectual property. If you would like permission to use material from the book (other than for review purposes), please contact permissions@hbgusa.com. Thank you for your support of the author's rights.

Grand Central Life & Style
Hachette Book Group
1290 Avenue of the Americas,
New York, NY 10104
grandcentrallifeandstyle.com
twitter.com/grandcentralpub

First Edition: March 2017

Grand Central Life & Style is an imprint of Grand Central Publishing. The Grand Central Life & Style name and logo are trademarks of Hachette Book Group, Inc.

The publisher is not responsible for websites (or their content) that are not owned by the publisher.

The Hachette Speakers Bureau provides a wide range of authors for speaking events. To find out more, go to www.hachettespeakersbureau.com or call (866) 376-6591.

Other photo credits: page 17 courtesy of Mesiyah McGinnis; pages 21 and 24 courtesy of Under Armour; page 25 courtesy of Daniil Simkin; pages 204 and 206 © 2014 Jacklyn Greenberg / JAGstudios; all other photos are from the author's personal collection.

Library of Congress Cataloging-in-Publication Data has been applied for.

ISBNs: 978-1-4555-9630-0 (hardcover),
978-1-4555-9631-7 (ebook),
978-1-5387-2802-4 (signed edition)

Printed in the United States of America

Q-MA

10 9 8 7 6 5 4 3 2 1

To all of us on this journey, working toward a healthier life
and happier heart, we are in this together.
I hope you all believe in yourselves every step of the way.
Know that every day is another opportunity
to keep trying. Work hard and know you're worth it.
Let's create our best versions of ourselves,
and the best versions of our ballerina bodies.

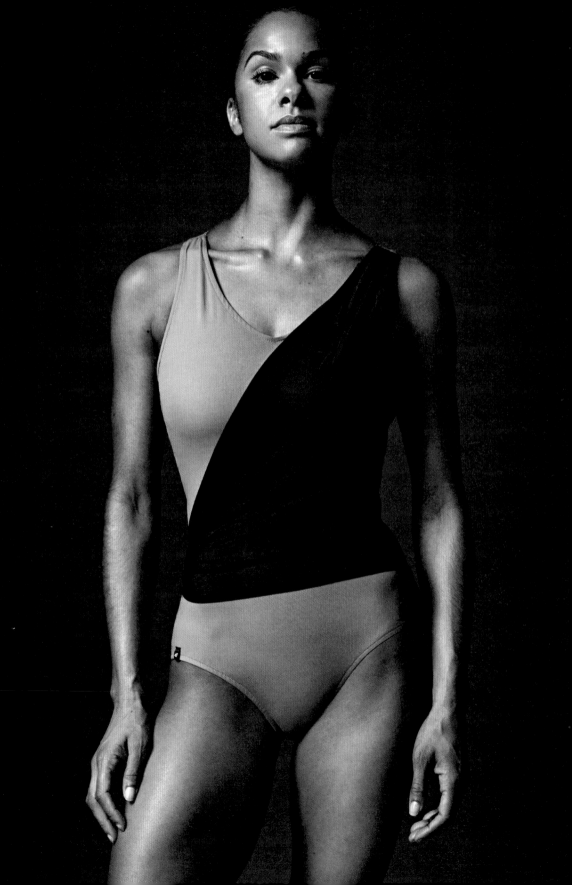

CONTENTS

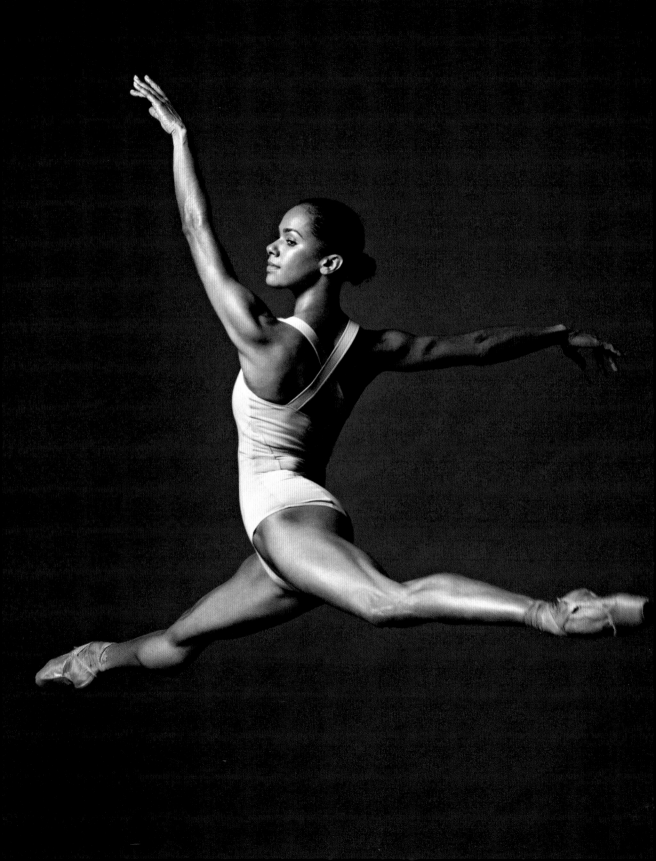

Still in Motion

spend countless hours at airports, particularly in the winter and summer months when American Ballet Theatre is on the road. While I'm waiting for the moment when it's finally time to board, I'll often stroll over to a newsstand and finger through the entertainment and fashion magazines lining the racks and shelves.

Cosmopolitan. Essence. Self. Peel back the covers and you can immerse yourself in worlds of beauty, fitness, and luxury. There are how-tos and what-fors; tips, diets, and schedules; an array of glossy blueprints that guide women on a path to a feminine ideal they are supposed to be striving for.

Without fail, the models or actresses who are featured are gorgeous, with luminous skin and lean physiques. When I was a young, naïve dancer, new to ABT and seeking my way, I was influenced and affected by those images. In my mind, I felt that this was what beauty was and I had to meet that standard. I struggled to figure out how I could maintain a healthy diet and lifestyle, not just on those days when I would be dining on room service, but also once I returned home to New York City.

I may have been an athlete, living in one of the world's most glamorous cities, but I had no nutritionist on speed dial, no extra money to hire a chef to prepare healthy meals. And while I was being taught the art of ballet daily, I wasn't getting the specific instruction I needed to keep every part of my body in peak shape.

I'd flip to the interviews in the magazine, searching for advice, eager to learn the featured celebrity's secrets. When asked how she stayed so taut, so fit, her answers would often be a riff on the same refrain. "I drink a lot of water! I get a lot of sleep! This is just me!"

To the young, insecure woman I was then, that explanation seemed impossibly simple. As the woman I have become, I know such advice makes up pieces of the puzzle, but it's hardly the whole solution. In recent years, I have had the honor of appearing in several magazines myself, and when reporters ask me what it's like to dance with one of the most prestigious ballet companies in the world, or what I eat to power through my regimen, or to stay strong and svelte, you know what I tell them? The truth.

None of it was easy. Not my climb in the ballet world, not my arrival at a place of personal contentment and peace, not my journey to the body I stand in.

When I was a child, my family often had little money, and we had to eat whatever we could afford. I used to love corn chips doused with hot sauce and glow-in-the-dark cheese squeezed out of a bottle.

Even after I'd become a dancer with ABT, putting my body through the rigors of dancing eight hours a day, five days a week, my body still craved meals that were heavy on the carbs because that was all it knew. And when my body bloomed in my late teens and I no longer fit the old-fashioned, pixie-like ballet ideal, I'd try to escape my frustration by diving into a box of sweets. I would eat every bite—and hate myself in the morning. In short, I understand the temptations, pressures, and frustrations of the real world.

I was an ordinary young woman, trying to determine what was best for my body, my health, my spirit, mostly on my own. Slowly, by experimenting, by adding cross-training to my schedule and tweaking my diet, I began to figure it out. I found what worked for me by trial and error. I learned that I couldn't do cardio that had weight training or too much resistance on the machines. I realized how to burn calories without adding bulk to my frame, and I discovered which cross-training helped me to strengthen my core and lengthen my muscles in a way that would not just benefit the structure of my body, but make me a stronger dancer as well. I discovered which foods gave me the fuel that my body needed after expending as much energy as I do every day.

I devised a plan for how to eat so that I could keep my body lean and powerful, and I realized that dietary discipline doesn't have to mean deprivation. Now I want to share all that I've learned with you.

I've always been a dreamer, and I am thankful that a lot of my dreams have come true, from becoming a professional ballet dancer to becoming the first African American principal ballerina in the history of American Ballet Theatre. Now I dream of sharing what I've learned—of showing women everywhere how to reach their body goals and achieve what they see as their best selves—using a ballerina body as the basis: one that is lean but sinewy, with muscles that are long, sculpted, and toned.

My regimen is grounded in the real world. Though my career involves constant exercise and dance, I know that not everyone has the time to make it to the gym each day. I'm a woman who as a child used a motel railing as a ballet barre, so I believe in the power of improvisation and being able to exercise right where you are. Your bedroom mattress can be your springboard; your natural body weight can be your ballast.

Change is not easy. It took years for me to find the balance of exercise and nutrition that worked best for my physique. But I also know from my personal experience that it's never too late to make change happen. Each morning, as the sun filters through your bedroom window and you wipe the sleep from your eyes, you can make a fresh start, you can rededicate yourself to your ongoing journey to take control of your body, your health, and your mental well-being.

We will take it one movement at a time, with a step-by-step guide that includes meal plans, workout routines, and words of inspiration to keep you motivated. You will eventually be able to mix and match foods on your own, but until you've found your own rhythm, you can refer to the twenty-one-day menu that I've created with plenty of options to keep you energized and satisfied.

Did you know fat is good for you? It's even better than that. It's great. And through meal plans and recipes that celebrate healthy fats and lean proteins, kicking your metabolism into shape, and a do-it-anywhere exercise plan that blends techniques from the worlds of ballet and floor barre, I will show women of every size and shape how they can become stronger and more vibrant, how they can feel their best so they can perform at their peak.

Ballerina Body is for women across the spectrum, from the college student trying to eat healthy and stay fit in the midst of dormitory life and exams, to the Gen Xer balancing her career with motherhood, to the retiree who wishes to stay active and healthy throughout her golden years.

My advice is based on what for me has been tried and true. It's modeled on how I have danced and lived, and it's rooted in the wisdom I have gleaned through my own errors and experimentation. You will likely experience your own trial and error along the way, but I'm sure that ultimately, your personal will and commitment will propel you toward success.

I know what it's like to deal with self-doubt, to feel it is an uphill battle to reach your goals. To many, I was too old and too brown to succeed in the rarefied and largely white world of ballet. But thanks to mentors who believed in me, hard work, and perseverance, I have been able to rise to the top tier of one of the world's premier ballet companies and to achieve a life balance that makes me feel centered and whole.

Just as there is a growing recognition that a ballerina's strength and grace can be embodied by a dancer of any hue, the idea of a ballerina's body has also been reshaped. It's no longer about looking childlike and brittle. We are real women *and* ballerinas, and we, as well as those who aspire to a similar physical ideal, want to be lean but also muscular, feminine but also strong, lithe but also curvaceous.

Ballerina Body provides a flexible and customizable road map that will help you maintain a healthy sense of your body as you attain optimal levels of strength, flexibility, and energy. While you may never perform grands jetés across the floorboards of a theater, my program will help guide you toward these goals:

- Strong, shapely legs and a toned derrière
- Youthful flexibility gained from the structure of a ballet class that combines strengthening and stretching exercises
- Crystal-cut curves all over your body
- A sexy fluidity and confidence wherever you go
- A new love for the body you have, and no more negative thoughts racing through your mind about what you look like
- A renewed physical and spiritual energy derived from careful, focused commitment to your best and strongest self
- A recognition of the importance of mentors in your life, to inspire, encourage, and motivate you for your journey, whether that's a quest for a healthy body, a new career, or simply a sense of inner contentment

Achieving your ballerina body will take commitment, work, and, yes, sacrifice. And just as your spirit, your personality, your natural shape, are all singular to you, each of your experiences with my program will also be unique. But there is enough flexibility in my plan to allow you to discover the mix of food, movement, and motivational exercises that works best for *you*. And while each of our journeys may differ slightly, the destination will be the same—a more vibrant body and emotional energy that will leave you feeling empowered, healthy, and whole.

So come on. We will get there. Together.

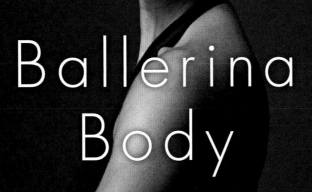

Ballerina
Body

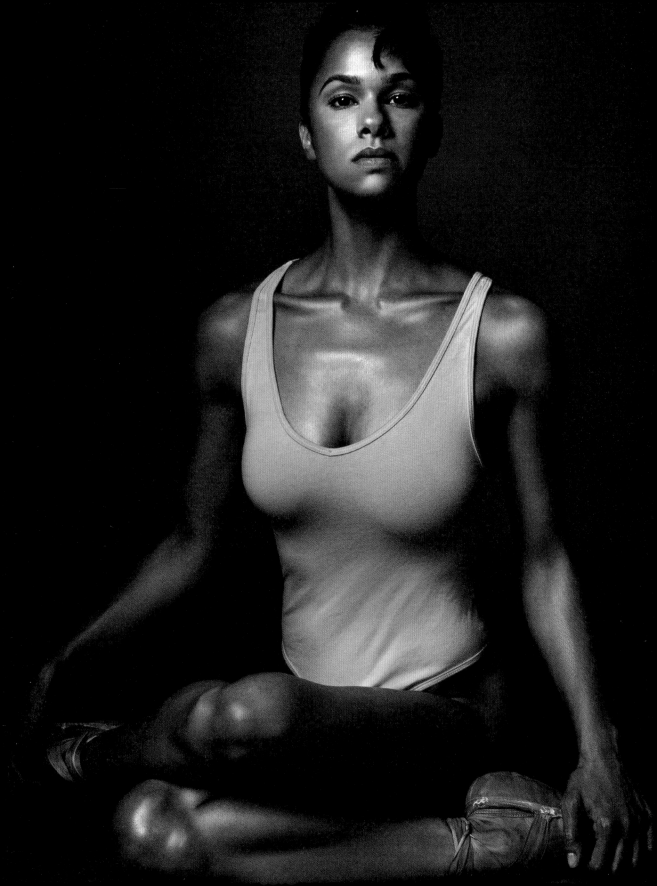

PART 1

Mind

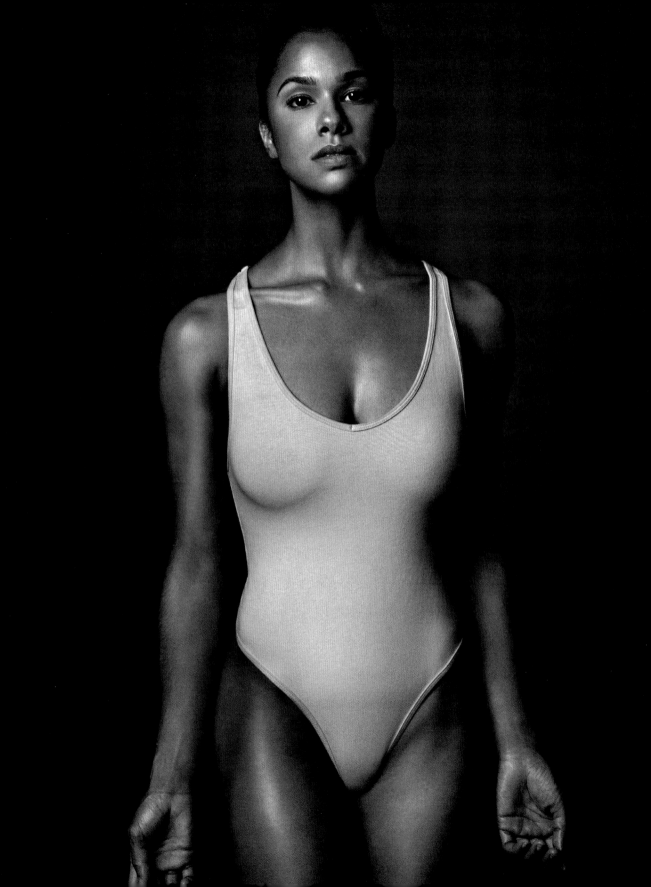

Chapter 1

YOUR BODY IS PERFECT FOR YOU

So much of my approach to my life and career stems from my experiences as a child. My need to please and be the best, my yearning for structure and discipline, all started back in Kansas City, Missouri, where I was born.

When I was a toddler, my family and I moved to the small West Coast city of Bellflower. There were four of us kids then: my older sister, Erica, my big brothers, Doug Jr. and Chris, and then me. My mother would marry two more times, and that's when my baby sister, Lindsey, and our baby brother, Cameron, would come along.

There was such a ruckus in our household, so many personalities clamoring for attention, that it was hard for me to find my own voice. It became little more than a whisper, tucked deep inside, and I shrank within myself.

Shy doesn't begin to describe how withdrawn I was. When I went to school, my heart would pound as I sat in class, dreading that I might be called on to answer a question or to offer my opinion. And I worried constantly, about being tardy, about making a mistake on a test, about doing something, anything, that would upset the people around me. When I was seven years old, I started to suffer from migraines, sometimes feeling so sick I'd have to leave school early and lie down in a pitch-black room until the pain and nausea faded away.

My mother had migraines as well, and they'd started for her when she was my age. But I believe that my searing headaches were also connected to the constant nervousness I felt dealing with the turbulence of the world around me.

Our family moved often, from one small, crowded apartment to another, before

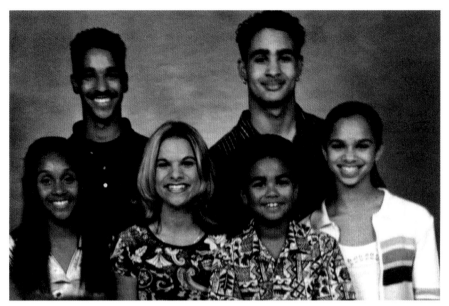

With my brothers and sisters; I'm on the right.

we finally landed at the Sunset Inn, a motel near a busy highway in the Southern California city of Gardena. So much upheaval, so much uncertainty, left me longing for stability and routine.

In the midst of all the chaos, music and movement were my refuge. Pliés and fouettés, the foundation of my future, were still over the horizon. I wasn't aware of ballet yet. I'd never even seen a ballet. Instead, I escaped to the rhymes and beats of rappers and singers like TLC, Salt-N-Pepa, and our family's favorite, Mariah Carey.

When I wasn't creating steps to the pop song of the moment, I was mimicking the moves of the legendary gymnast Nadia Comaneci. I'd seen a Lifetime movie based on her life story and I fell in love with her fierceness and grace. I began to teach myself the moves that she performed so effortlessly, and I found that I, too, could execute a cartwheel or the splits with ease.

But it was ballet that would be my calling, and my salvation. And I found it on the sweat-stained floor of a Boys & Girls Club gym. Every day, after school and drill team practice, I would head with my siblings to the local Boys & Girls Club, an organization that gave countless children like me a welcoming space to play and grow. Elizabeth Cantine, my drill team instructor and a woman whom I, to this day, consider my godmother, saw the way I moved and suggested that I attend a ballet class at the club, which was taught by a friend of hers, Cynthia Bradley.

As I've said, I didn't have a clue about ballet. And when I made my way to the bleachers to sit and watch Cynthia teach a handful of students how to stretch and pirouette, I felt even more lost. Trying something new, in a group of strangers, was terrifying to a shy, cautious child like me.

But Cynthia spotted me sitting there and gently encouraged me to join the group. I didn't even have a pair of tights or a leotard. It took a few days more for me to summon my courage, but, finally, with gym shorts that were too big, and socks barely topping my ankles, I walked across the floor, joined the class, and put my hands on the barre.

I was thirteen, far too old in the eyes of many purists to be getting my start in ballet. But with that first class, I'd brushed up against my destiny.

———

"You're too big to be a ballerina."

That's what a random stranger said to me one night, several years ago, at a Manhattan club. His words stopped me cold and sent a jagged pain through my heart.

I was in my second year in ABT's corps de ballet, the large group of dancers who create the atmosphere for the ballet and who frame the soloists and principal dancers who headline the performances. My best friend, Leyla, and I had taken a cab that evening to hang out at a popular new club called Bed. It was the kind of place where after spinning on the dance floor, partiers lounged on couches, chatted over the DJ's swelling beats, and sipped cocktails.

I'd gone to the club to forget what had happened a few hours before. But that stranger's callous comment brought roaring back the memory of everything I'd experienced that day, along with my feelings of confusion and even despair.

That afternoon, members of ABT's staff said they wanted to speak to me, and I had a good idea what they wanted to talk about. I'd put on ten pounds. My breasts pulled at the seams of the costumes I shared with my dance mates and wore as one of the Willies in *Giselle* and as a cygnet in *Swan Lake*. It was as if I was now enveloped in someone else's body.

The changes in my figure had happened seemingly overnight. A couple of years before, at nineteen years old, I'd had a physique more akin to that of a prepubescent girl. My doctor had grown concerned about my ability to maintain the strength I needed for my strenuous dance schedule, so he prescribed birth control pills to help my body catch up to where biologically it should have already been.

Of course, over time, my ballet instructors noticed the change. So that afternoon, when they called me in, they told me gently but firmly that I needed to "lengthen." In the ballet world, that was a polite way of saying that I needed to slim down.

Their admonishment stung, just like the words uttered by that man at the club. I

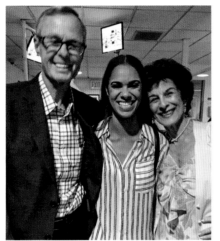
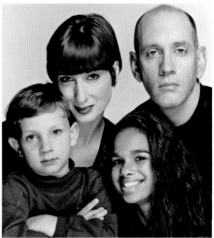

With Dick and Elizabeth Cantine.

With Cynthia Bradley and her family.

felt helpless. How was I going to lose weight? Where would I begin? I already spent up to eight hours a day rehearsing and taking ballet classes. During the season I performed several days a week. How could that not be enough? I needed nourishment to power through my classes and rehearsals. And at the end of a long day, I enjoyed a good meal, maybe even dessert. Did I now have to count every calorie and deny myself the occasional sweet treat? I was dejected. But as tough as those words were to hear, that conversation with my instructors at ABT, and the harsh realization that flowed from it, marked the true beginning of my fitness journey.

My path mirrored the rocky start of so many women. First you want to fit into a certain mold. Then you struggle to create or find a road map to get there. What I learned during my personal odyssey was sometimes painful, sometimes difficult, but always invaluable. No, I didn't have to lock my refrigerator and throw away the key, but I did need to eat more mindfully so that I could build my strength and give myself the breathing room for that occasional dessert or glass of wine. No, I didn't have to lift heavy weights and work out around the clock. But I had to learn what exercises and combinations of foods would keep my body lean and strong and give me the stamina I needed to get through my long days.

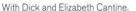

It took me a few years to get the formula exactly right. But when I did, not only did I feel fitter, not only was my body sleeker and more powerful, but I also had come to a realization that was more important than any other—I came to understand, to accept, that all along my body had been *perfect* for me.

My body *was* and *is* perfect for me, just like the body you're in is perfect for you. Didn't it pop out of bed when it was still dark outside and hold you up through homeroom, algebra, and band rehearsal after school? Didn't it carry you across the campus quad, through your procession of classes, and then forward, until you headed home from your part-time job? Didn't it carry your twins for nine long months and then usher them into the world? Hasn't your body held you in good stead through the decades, and isn't it sustaining you now in middle age?

Like I said. You are *perfect*.

You may have to start fueling your body differently so that you can climb the stairs without losing your breath. You may have to strengthen your core so your bearing is as regal as you are. You may need to incorporate some physical rituals that can help you feel more alert when you hit that midway point in the afternoon, or reframe your thinking so you can enter that marathon and run it to the end.

But that doesn't mean there's anything *wrong* with the body you're in, that your physique should be a replica of your favorite singer's, athlete's, or movie star's. It just means fine-tuning, tweaking, honing, what you've already got, taking control of and subtly re-etching the outer self that is divinely *you*.

How boring would it be if we all looked the same? No, really. Just as it would be monotonous, off-putting, and surreal for us all to have the same hair color, eye tint, and shade of skin, we are also not all meant to be exactly the same size.

I actually think fixating on numbers, whether they appear on the tag stitched to the back of your blouse, the scale that sits on your bathroom floor, or a sheet of paper where you painstakingly track the calories in every meal, is not the most productive path toward your healthiest self. The fit of your clothing, the vibrancy of your complexion, the intensity of your energy, are all, in my mind, better gauges of whether or not you are boosting your vitality and performing at your peak.

To be sure, many of the messages echoing through our culture make some women feel that we are all supposed to fit into the same waifish, cookie-cutter mold. Even dancers, often in top shape because of the grueling workouts we put our bodies through, have plenty of insecurities. After all, we spend a good part of our day in front of mirrors. Add to that the pressures of being judged by dance instructors, critics, and, most important, the audience, and it can make even the most confident performer feel tentative and unsure. But even those who do not spend chunks of their lives beneath a spotlight can feel self-conscious about their figures.

You don't need to internalize someone else's rendering of what it means to be beautiful and healthy. Rather than comparing yourself to photographs in a magazine or images on a television screen, the only visage you need to focus on is the one that stares back at you from your own mirror. And thankfully women are starting to rebel against limited and unrealistic notions of what it is to be attractive and are instead embracing their own unique beauty.

The mental snapshot of a ballerina's body has also changed. Women are flocking to barre workouts taught at studios and gyms like Pure Barre, the Dailey Method, and Equinox because they want to be willowy but not fragile, toned but not tiny, muscular but not masculine. They understand that the perfect body is one that is robust and healthy.

––––––––––

Sometimes we turn to strict diets to try to attain the body we desire. But dieting is often an ephemeral fix, rather than a long-term, sustainable solution. You can carve out the physique and lifestyle you want without limiting yourself to a handful of foods or severely restricting your calories. The healthier way to achieve your goals is by adjusting your lifestyle bit by bit, incorporating subtle changes that you can then commit to and live by.

I eventually realized there was nothing wrong with the natural changes that my body had undergone, but I had to learn to work with this new physique, to find the exercise techniques it needed to push through hours upon hours of rehearsal. I had to learn to listen to this new body, to know what nutrition it required to fuel performances that required sheer athleticism blended with a dancer's grace. I had to embrace my new physical self to attain my goals of maximum health and vigor.

As a dancer, my body is my instrument. I speak to the audience through every muscle and tendon, with every glissade and renversé. When I recognized those truths, my fitness journey became one of joy and not frustration. I wanted simply to respect my body, to get the most out of it that I could, in order to live my best life.

Your body is essential to you as well. That's why it's so important to love it, to have faith in it. Take a stack of sticky notes and paste reminders of all it does for you all over your mirror, or jot words of appreciation on the lined pages of your journal—*My legs propelled me out of bed this morning. These shoulders gave a piggyback ride to my children. My arms allowed me to rake the soil in my garden on a Sunday afternoon.*

There have been times when I doubted myself, questioning if I had what it took to advance from a member of the corps de ballet to soloist, and then, one day, to principal. I had many days when I thought I'd never master the mix of exercise and food that would help me maximize my endurance and effectiveness as a dancer. But an endless loop of self-doubt chips away at our feelings of self-worth, stifling our motivation and crippling our momentum before we take even our first step.

So, let the first act of our fitness journey start from a place of self-respect and appreciation. We want to polish the bodies that are our temples, not tear them down.

When negative thoughts rise in your mind and start to go round and round—*My stomach is too jiggly! My thighs are too wobbly! My arms are too flabby!*—push those self-critiques away and refocus on how singular you are, and how, with small changes and small efforts each and every day, you can become stronger, more vibrant, more sculpted, no matter what your natural shape.

By shifting my focus, changing my self-perception, and shoring up my spirituality, I have come to love the body that I am in. The muscles that ripple through my legs allow me to do thirty-two fouettés without crumpling to the floor. The curves that swell beneath my clothes help me to relay the message to the world that you can be healthy, fit, and, yes, voluptuous too. My physique, like the color of my skin, is helping people reconsider what a ballerina looks like.

You are fiercely, lovingly, and divinely *you*. My ballet-based fitness plan is simply going to help you maximize the wonderful body that you already have and enable you to be as fit, joyful, and dynamic as you can possibly be.

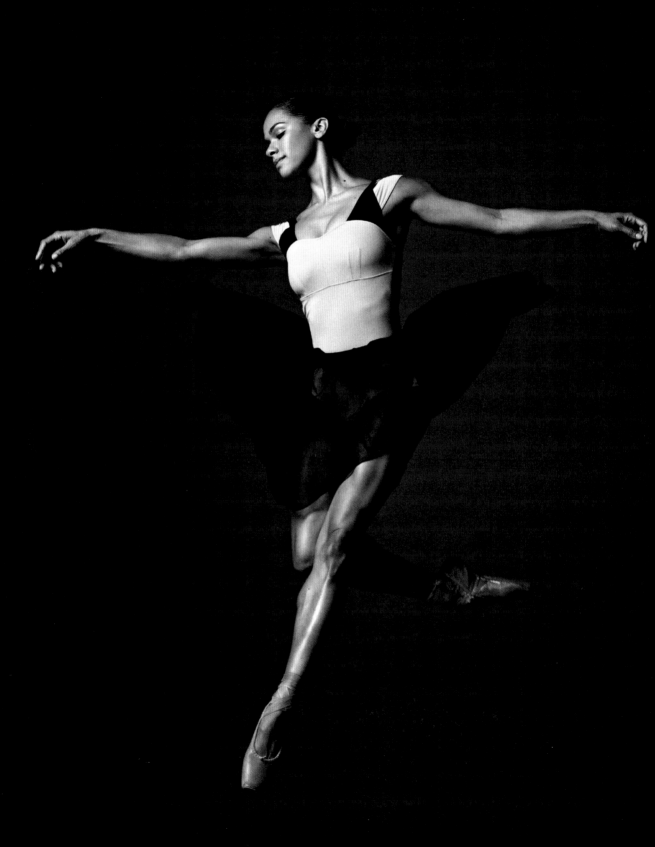

Chapter 2

GET INSPIRED

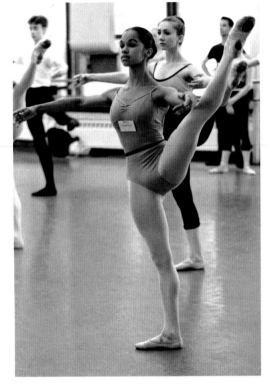

've wanted to dance for American Ballet Theatre since I was thirteen years old.

ABT became my beacon when I first saw videos of Mikhail Baryshnikov and Gelsey Kirkland, two of its most legendary dancers, perform. I held on to that dream when I attended my first summer intensive program with the San Francisco Ballet, receiving training to help bring more clarity and strength to my technique. And every time I strained a muscle or crashed to the floor while attempting a new turn or leap, the goal of dancing with ABT gave me the power to keep going.

Whether we realize it or not, each of us sets goals, markers that we aim for, every day. They can often be routine, like when we set the alarm because we have the intention of getting up at a certain time. Or our goals can have a payoff that looms far in the distance, like when we funnel a few dollars into a savings account to seed a rainy-day fund, or do research on a destination that we hope to one day visit.

GOALS: KEEPING A FINISH LINE IN SIGHT

Goals are essential. If you don't have clarity about what you want to accomplish, you can't plot how you will get there. And all of us need a spark to keep us energized and on task when we have those inevitable moments of feeling weary or discouraged. A strong emotional foundation can keep you invigorated, while having a finish line in sight, a target to aim for, can help you harness the mental energy and focus you need to reach it.

It's important to remember that we don't have to achieve whatever we are seeking in one mighty leap. That's overwhelming—and unrealistic. Instead, we can move forward in the direction of our ultimate goal, one small step, one tiny victory, at a time. Achieving the strength and figure you desire begins with that first morning that you will yourself to work out when you'd rather lie in bed an extra half hour. You move closer every time you skip the fast food and prepare a healthier home-cooked meal instead. Or when you leave your car in the garage and take an energizing walk to the dry cleaners or grocery store.

I used to imagine myself standing in ABT's studio at 890 Broadway in Manhattan. I declared that I would be there when I said good-bye at the end of summer in San Francisco to a good friend who had the same dream. In 1998, when I was sixteen, I tried out for and earned a spot in ABT's summer intensive program. It was the first significant milestone in what would be a long, sometimes difficult, professional journey. But I had reached my goal.

―――――

As you move toward your ballerina body, you aren't just stripping away calories; you are embracing a whole new lifestyle that will transform the way you eat, the way you work out, and how you feel. Those are changes that won't happen in an instant. Along the path to better fitness and nutrition, there will be plenty of messages that threaten to pull you off track, from the barrage of commercials advertising a new pizza topping or chocolate treat that causes your stomach to rumble just before bedtime, to the ubiquitous diet programs that promise a menu or plan that will allow you to eat your way to the body of your dreams—for a small fee.

When you have aspirations—the goal to sculpt a more limber and powerful physique, the determination to be able to skip the escalator and bound up the steps instead—your own mental messaging can help drown out all the distracting outside chatter. You can create your own internal sound track to motivate and root you on.

Decide what you want. *Declare* it to the world. *See* yourself winning. And remember that if you are persistent as well as patient, you can get whatever you seek.

MOTIVATION: A GOAL BEYOND YOURSELF

You're worth it. None of your effort, not a minute of your time, is wasted as you strive toward becoming your best, most vibrant self. But sometimes, as sisters, mothers, partners, friends, we feel guilty taking our attention off of others. You should never feel unworthy of self-nurturing, but in case you do, remember this truth: When we achieve our own dreams, we carry others with us.

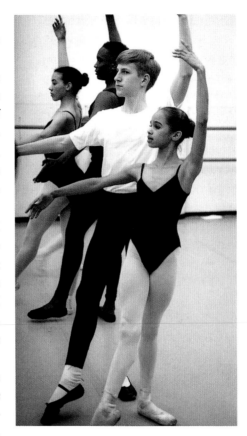

I knew from the first time I touched the barre in that San Pedro gym that ballet was what I was meant to do. I was an anxious child, but when I danced I felt a burst of confidence. I was a shy girl, unsure of my own voice, but I felt I was able to communicate with the world through ballet.

My career climb was rapid, from starting to dance at the relatively late age of thirteen, to becoming an apprentice with ABT just four years later, to joining ABT's studio company soon after. At nineteen, I got promoted to the main company's corps de ballet. I'd checked off one goal after another.

But once I was part of the corps, I started to feel unsure about whether I would be able to grab hold of the next brass ring—becoming a soloist and, eventually, a principal. I suffered an injury early on that left me sidelined for a year. When I recovered and returned to dancing, I was told that my new, curvier figure was no longer ideal. And at times I felt isolated and underestimated because of the color of my skin.

At one point, I contemplated leaving ABT. I was offered a soloist position with the Dance Theatre of Harlem, a diverse company filled with talented dancers where I believed the spotlight would be on my ability and not my skin color.

But as appealing as the idea seemed, I knew that I would never be fulfilled by that decision; ABT was my dream. I turned that opportunity down. I wanted to succeed at ABT, and I realized my dream had to do with far more people than me.

Having a mission beyond yourself can sometimes give you the boost you need to hold fast and keep pushing toward your goal. In my own life, the belief that I wasn't dancing just for myself, but for all the black ballerinas who had come before me and not gotten the opportunities their artistry deserved, convinced me to stay at ABT and continue striving. When my confidence faltered, I thought of the children I wanted to encourage, girls and boys with backgrounds like mine, who'd perhaps never envisioned a career in classical dance because of their ethnicity or socioeconomic background, and I became determined to show them what was possible.

On your quest to achieve a ballerina body, think about all the reasons that you want it. If you simply want to be your healthiest self, that's reason enough. But perhaps you also aspire to be able to play an active role in your grandchildren's lives for years to come. You may be craving extra energy to pour into your business, and that professional kick start can enable you to provide jobs in your community. You may want to succeed on your wellness journey just to show yourself you can. But your victory could also inspire others to go after their own ambitions.

Every action we take begins with a thought. You may want a more powerful physique to give you the energy to help others, or more vigor in your mind, spirit, and body to propel you toward attaining even more of your dreams. Whatever your motivations, once you have conceived them in your mind, say them out loud to your friends, to your loved ones, or simply to yourself. Tap the words into your smartphone, or write them on a piece of paper and tape it to your bathroom mirror.

Now that you know what you want and why you want it, you need to have faith that with time and determination, you can achieve it. *Picture* the results. *Envision* the outcome. *Imagine* that you have won—even before you've engaged in your first workout.

VISUALIZATION: SEEING IS ACHIEVING

Visualization, seeing ourselves victorious in whatever endeavor we take on, is one of the most powerful tools that we have in our mental and emotional arsenal. Athletes often tap into that strategy. Tiger Woods has said that he would visualize how a ball would travel through the air and then how it would land on the putting green before he took a shot. U.S. women's soccer champion Carli Lloyd has spoken often about how she imagines her feats on the field long before she gets there.

Your mind's eye is truly powerful. Envisioning that you have already arrived wherever you want to be can elevate your confidence, enhance your concentration, and help your muscles to fire on all cylinders.

In 2012, I experienced one of the highlights of my career when I starred in Igor Stravinsky's *The Firebird* at the Metropolitan Opera House. But that first performance was also my last in the role that season—and potentially, the final act of my career.

I'd injured my leg months earlier, but I kept up a grueling schedule of rehearsals and performances on the road to make sure I was prepared for my *Firebird* debut at the Met. When I couldn't take the pain any longer and went to the doctor, I learned I'd suffered six stress fractures in my tibia, a large bone that lies below the knee.

Dancers often get hurt dancing, jumping, training, and performing for hours on end. I'd had stress fractures before. But this was the most serious injury I'd ever suffered. I soon had a major operation in which a plate was put in my leg. I didn't know what my future held. But I *did* know that I couldn't allow the ballerina in me to die. I had to summon all the mental and emotional strength I could muster to keep my inner fire going. I could barely walk, let alone dance, but I began to visualize myself healed. And I danced inside my head.

Each morning, when you wake up, or whenever you can carve out a quiet moment in your day, I'd like you to pause for a few minutes to paint a mental picture. Catch a glimpse of your elegant gait as you stroll by a store window. Envision your chiseled legs rippling beneath your dress on a bright summer day. Feel the bounce in your step as you head to a meeting. Bask in a warm breeze as you stay present in the moment, no longer consumed with negative thoughts about your body or your appearance. Seeing is believing—*and* achieving.

After my injury, I worked out every morning with my instructor Marjorie Liebert, who was trained in the floor barre technique known as Kniaseff barre-à-terre, a way of movement that we will draw on to help you shape your ballerina body. Those exercises allowed me to execute moves I would normally have done standing at the barre, while lying down on my living room floor.

I would lie on my stomach, my back, my sides, and imagine myself upright, "on my leg," dancing. Looking up at the ceiling, gently lifting my arms above my head to practice my port de bras, I would see myself on the stage, executing fouettés, jumping in *Les Sylphides*. I worked on strengthening my core, my back, my legs, all the while envisioning myself already back at ABT, stronger, more graceful, a better dancer than I'd been before.

Not only did my physical exercises keep my body primed so that when I was able to return to ballet class my muscles retained the memory of what they needed to do; I believe that visualizing myself whole and healed sped up my recovery. The images inside my head kept me focused and dedicated, giving me the stamina to keep working and helping me to block out the depression and fear that could have stopped me cold.

If you can manifest what you want mentally, you can achieve it physically. I have learned from personal experience that our emotional selves are so much stronger than we know.

KEEP A JOURNAL: PUT PEN TO PAPER

When I found ballet, I found a way to channel my voice for the first time. It had always been difficult for me to express myself, and dance emboldened me, allowing me to speak through the power of motion. But when it came to actual words, I still struggled—until I was fifteen and discovered that I could articulate my aspirations, my emotions, in the pages of a journal.

Keeping a journal can be a great way for you to chart your progress toward your ballerina body. Your journal is your refuge, a private space where you can pour out all your thoughts and feelings. You want it to feel special, so maybe designate a certain pen that you don't use for anything else, and a chair, a corner, or a room that can become a cocoon where you curl up and write.

Then, when you are ready, start with your beginning—how you look and feel now, and how you want to look and feel at the end of your journey—along with all of the reasons you're embarking on this quest for mental and physical fitness.

If you are struggling some evenings to stay on track with your meal plan or workout, write it down. Then pull back, think about the roadblocks, and write those down too. Did you feel that your schedule was too jam-packed to exercise today? Were the bar snacks and chocolate cake too hard to resist when you went out last night with your friends? Are you just plain frustrated that the image in your mirror isn't transforming fast enough, and so for a moment you felt like giving up?

And what about that morning when you pushed yourself further than you thought you could go? When you didn't feel like working out, but you changed into your leggings, grabbed your towel, and did it anyway? Write it *all* down. It will offer you insight.

Putting pen to paper proved cathartic for me. Seeing my goals, my thoughts, my experiences, jotted in vivid detail helped me to gain perspective on all that I was going through, as well as chronicle my life's journey on and off the stage.

A Picture Is Worth a Thousand Words—Creating a Vision Board

A vision board is a kind of aspirational collage. Whether you're aiming for straight As at the end of the semester, a promotion at work, or your new ballerina body and lifestyle, it's taking the goal you visualize in your head, or the vision you've articulated in your journal, and translating it into a collection of images. That way you have another, ever-present reminder of what you're aiming for, giving you an energy boost when your confidence lags, and inspiring you along your path.

Don't tuck it in a corner. Put it in a space where you'll pass it every day, maybe next to your computer, your TV, or the spot where you charge your phone. And make it a reflection of you. Your quotes can be scrawled like graffiti or clipped from a magazine. Tack up postcards and photographs, and choose patterns and colors that invigorate you or, if you prefer, those that quiet your mind. This is a vehicle for your creativity and aspiration, and yet another means for staying focused and motivated. We can never have too many.

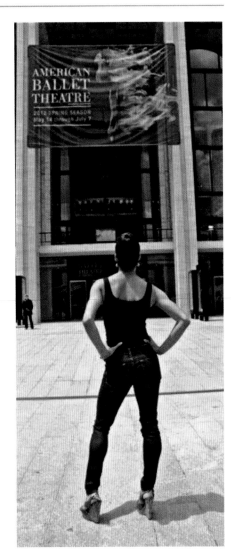

Transformation is hard. Transformation takes time. We're not trying out a magical fad that will lead to quick-to-fade results. We are carving out a new approach to living, a holistic way of eating, exercising, and thinking. As you tweak your diet and build on your fitness routine, dramatic physical change may not show up right away, and that can make it hard to recognize all that you are accomplishing.

That's why documenting your journey, the steps that move you forward as well as those that sometimes set you back, can be so empowering. You're constantly reminded of your mission, all the reasons you took it on, and all of your momentum, however incremental it may sometimes seem.

In my own life, I know that being able to go back and read entries from the past has helped me learn about the woman I am becoming by gaining insights into the person I have been. I've written down my most exhilarating moments, as well as my biggest fears and disappointments. I still journal. This is what I wrote not long after I learned I had been promoted to principal dancer in 2015.

> *This doesn't feel real. Overwhelming. I just want to work, especially in times like this when I'm being celebrated and criticized, even though I've reached an unbelievable goal. I get criticism because very few dancers have reached this level of success. I think they wonder, Why me? People say I'm a fraud, that I just want the fame. When I see things like that written, I tend to go to that place of, "Who am I? Am I the real deal? Am I good enough?" Maybe in a couple of months it will sink in.*

Rereading that passage a few months later, I realized that it *had* begun to sink in, that I'd gained some valuable perspective. I knew that I couldn't pretend that my insecurities had disappeared. But I also knew that when those feelings came up, I had to quickly let them go. Having wanted this opportunity my entire career, now that I was here, I had to have patience with myself, to take the time to find my footing and make this new position my own. I didn't need to be any other dancer—not the ballerina dancing beside me or anyone who had come before; I just needed to be *me*. And I am good enough.

You are good enough. Sometimes you may doubt yourself. Maybe you've dieted in the past, only to see the results you fought so hard for disappear when you returned to your old routine. You may have had the best of intentions when you bought your gym membership but soon realized it was wasted because you rarely found the time to get there. You may need a little time to make the Ballerina Body program your own, to find your footing as you adopt a new way of living, but don't compare yourself to anyone else! Find the pace, the schedule, the meal and workout combinations, that work best for *you*.

By keeping in touch with yourself through journaling, you will have a written record of what does and doesn't work for your body. You can turn to your own personal reflections for encouragement. You'll be able to measure, with your own words, your own trial and error, how much progress you've made on your unique journey, and ultimately, how much you have grown.

Say It Like You Mean It— Affirming the Results You Want to See

In addition to seeing yourself where you want to be, putting that vision into words is also a way to bring it into being. You are making a declaration to yourself.

I am worthy. I am strong.

I think it's best to start your mornings with an affirmation, but you can speak it at the end of the day or whenever you have a few quiet moments. Just try to do it at the same time every day to create a rhythm, a designated point in the day when you make a promise to yourself.

You can read the words in your journal or say them out loud while gazing in the mirror. Remember, don't ask a question or make a plea. Say it like you mean it.

I am healthy. I am joyful. I am victorious.

I think it's also a good idea to offer up a few words of gratitude every day. There are so many things in life that we have to be thankful for, though we don't always think about them in that way, whether it's sharing a laugh with your friends after school, getting a text from someone you have missed and not seen in a long time, or seeing the sun rise.

Think about starting or ending each journal entry with expressions of gratitude for your body, for the people you love who are in your life, for the hobbies and pursuits that fill you with passion.

I am thankful that I woke up this morning and get to enjoy another day! I am grateful for my newfound strength! I appreciate my loved ones who are just a phone call away!

Showing appreciation for the many, many gifts in our lives helps us to take joy in the moment, to not let the preciousness of life just pass us by. And it reminds us that we already have more than enough. The goals that we aim for, and reach, are just a wonderful bonus.

SLOW AND STEADY WINS THE RACE

Setting small, incremental goals makes our journey to wellness more manageable. Our confidence grows every time we reach a new milestone, reminding us that we really do have the power to achieve whatever we desire.

Still, we all have moments when we feel tired or grow impatient. We may want to give up if we're not seeing the results that we want as fast as we would like. But having a mission beyond yourself can keep you motivated: *I'm not just doing this for me. I want to be my healthiest self for my family, for my community, for the young people who may look up to me!*

See yourself vibrant and strong, emotionally centered and healthy. Write down your biggest challenges and your smallest victories. Being able to reflect on all you've overcome, as well as all that you have achieved, will make your ultimate triumph even sweeter.

Mindfulness and centeredness have been key to my success and have enabled me to overcome many personal setbacks. Becoming your fittest, most vibrant, empowered self will not happen overnight. But being clear about your goals, envisioning how great and confident you'll feel, and chronicling your feelings, experiences, and successes along the way will give you the jolt you need to keep working, to keep reaching, to keep pushing, all the way to the finish line.

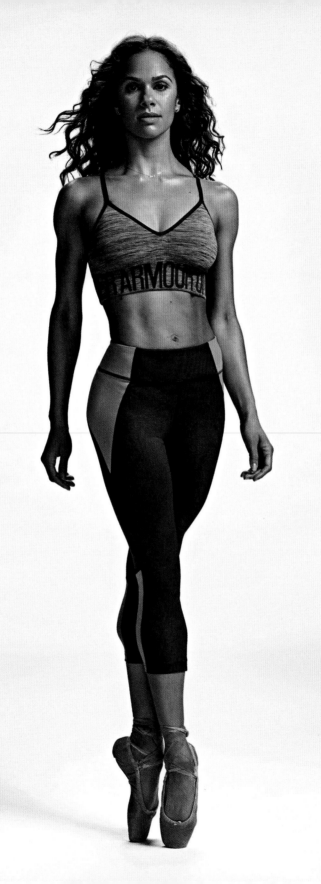

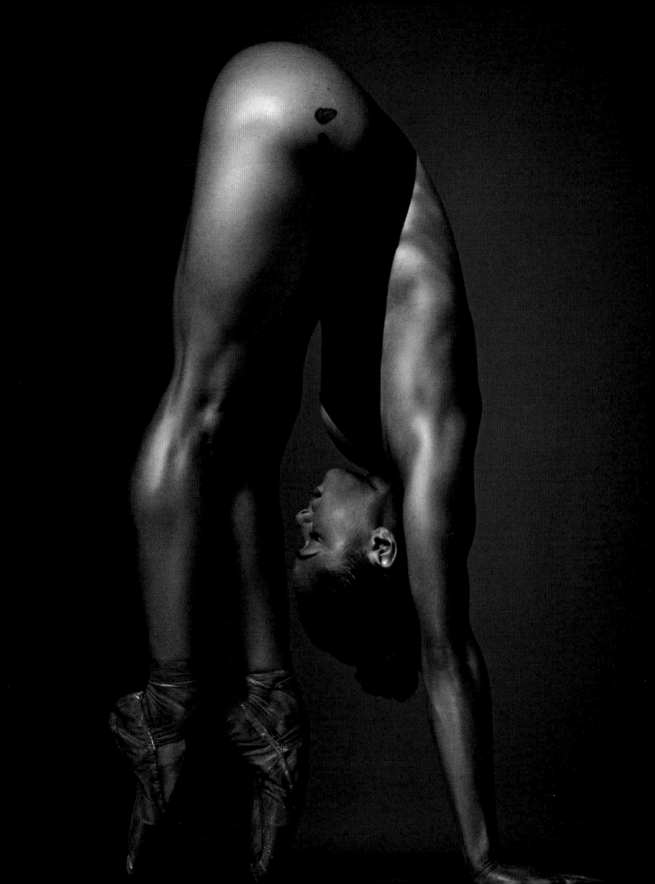

Chapter 3

BALANCE: FINDING INNER PEACE

t can take years before a young ballerina is able to stand en pointe, rising on her toes and then holding firm for seconds or even minutes. To accomplish that feat she must find the strength, possess the dexterity, master the balance.

Balance, so central to ballet, is even more crucial in life. Our minds, bodies, and spirits are intricately connected, and we are our best selves when all are in sync.

We need mental focus to take action, whether that's solving a problem at work or deciding to reshape our physiques. We need to fuel our bodies with the best nutrition to maximize our energy. And being mentally grounded can give us strength beyond the physical. Being in tune with our inner selves, as well as the broader natural order that exists all around us, keeps us steady in the midst of life's many challenges and unleashes the inner resolve that can help us accomplish each of our goals.

FINDING INNER BALANCE: RITUAL

One of the key ways to access our inner power and balance is through ritual, those gestures we repeatedly turn to in order to calm ourselves, to help us cope, or to give us the fortitude to conquer a particular task. It can be the prayer you whisper every time you are about to board a flight, the deep breaths that you take to slow your pounding heart before a presentation, the "lucky" pin you attach to your blouse whenever you perform, or the affirmation that you recite before taking each of your final exams or

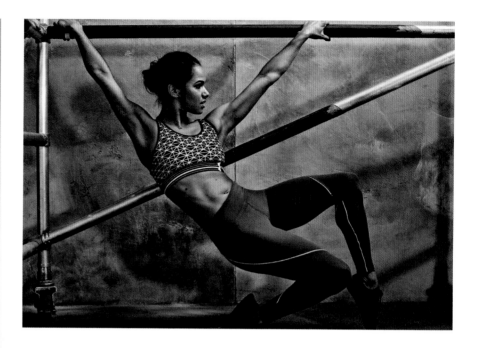

want to reach or a chore that we have to do, rituals can also positively affect the outcome by calming our anxieties and boosting our confidence.

Rituals can be rooted in religion—rubbing the rosary, chanting in front of a Buddhist *gohonzon*—or grounded in superstition. (Before we dancers take the stage, we often yell out *merde*, a bit of French slang that doesn't translate as "break a leg" but is meant to have the same effect—wishing the best of luck without tempting fate.) But rituals can also emerge from the simplest, the most mundane, of routines.

When I am about to perform, the hour that I spend in the dressing room applying my makeup and doing my hair helps to settle and soothe my mind. I close out the world around me, putting in my earphones and turning up the volume on my iPhone. Then I turn my attention to the brushes, tubes, and compacts laid out on the dressing room vanity, and as I powder my face and color my cheeks, I slow my breathing and focus on the piece I am about to dance.

That ritual, as much a part of my performing life as ballet class or rehearsal, takes me away from all the motion swirling around me backstage and the thoughts racing through my head. It gives me time for quiet reflection and allows me to focus on what I need to do onstage. I get the mental boost I need to believe that what I envision— giving a strong performance—will become a reality.

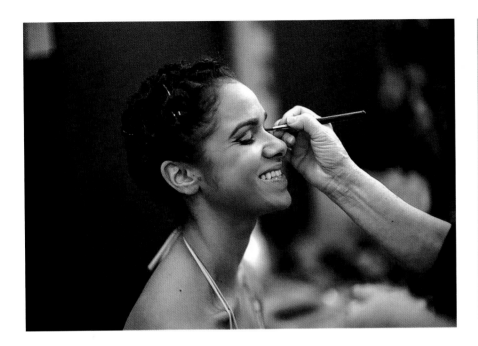

TAP INTO YOUR INTUITIVE POWER

We all have a well of inner resolve that we can draw on whenever we need it, an intuition that guides us if we just take the time to listen. Finding ways to tap into that power is vital. You can increase your self-awareness by engaging in actual meditation (see sidebar, page 28), or you can delve more deeply into any activity that gives you peace. Take what you already enjoy and then deepen the experience to better hear your inner voice and enhance your feelings of well-being.

If drawing puts you at ease, the next time you sit down with a sketch pad and pencil, take a few deep breaths to calm yourself. Then, instead of trying to conjure what you will sketch in your mind, let your intuitive self take over, guiding your hand and creating your work.

Or maybe you are musical. Instead of approaching your instrument with the determination to practice or learn a new song, try not to concentrate on a single note. Focus instead on the feel of the guitar strings pulling at your fingers, the echoing of the chords, the free flow of the melody. Get in the moment, and stay there, simply enjoying the experience of giving life to music.

Whatever your individual passions, something that we can all do is simply sit and be still. But instead of closing your eyes, as you would to meditate, keep them wide open and take in the wonder around you. When we are present and open to our environment, we also open up and awaken to our inner selves. Suddenly, the answer to that vexing problem may become crystal clear. That situation that seems overwhelming may appear less daunting. With stillness can come clarity.

Sometimes life changes because of our own initiative, like your decision to transform your workout routine to attain a ballerina body. But we all know that life can also evolve in ways beyond our control. Rituals provide a respite, a bit of stability in the midst of change, and they give you the opportunity to recalibrate whenever you need it—to check in with yourself, quiet your mind, and, for a little while, just be.

MOVING FOR THE JOY OF IT

We're going to embark on a whole regimen of exercise to create your ballerina body, strengthening your core, lengthening and defining your muscles, and ultimately giving a giant boost to your health. I hope you will engage in every move with enthusiasm, appreciating the payoff that's coming and how great you will feel. But your fitness journey will take dedication, it will take effort, and that won't feel like a romp at the beach.

Yet movement can be playful. When we are in motion, our imaginations can run free, our lungs fill with fresh air, and we become aware of our life-affirming heartbeat. There are actual chemical changes that occur in our bodies, making us feel more at peace. So along with the exercises that you will engage in for the purpose of gaining strength and staying fit, I believe it's important to find forms of movement that you do just for the joy of it.

Take a moment to reflect on activities that make you happy, actions that you don't think of as chores. Are your spirits lifted when you are out walking your dog? Do you feel calm when you're riding your bike around campus, or exhilarated when you're picking up speed on a hoverboard? Once you figure out what you purely enjoy, make the time to get in motion, even if it's for just half an hour each day.

Ballet has been my safe haven, an art form that allows me to create, imagine, and escape. To this day, even though ballet is my job, my career, the studio is still where I find time for quiet reflection.

Every morning I take ballet class. It's necessary even after all these years so that I can maintain my technique and keep my body primed to perform. But that hour and a half every day is also a form of meditation for me and my fellow dancers. It's a routine, familiar and constant, that our bodies and minds have come to crave and rely on. It's our chance to reset and prepare, so that we feel strong and ready for whatever the day may bring, whether that's eight hours of rehearsals, a performance that afternoon, or all of our other responsibilities that have nothing to do with dance.

When I was a child, ballet class gave me a reprieve from the chaos of my home life, and as a grown woman I still feel that that time grants me a little distance from all the other things jotted on my calendar, whether it's whittling the invitation list for my wedding or answering my emails. I actually asked my wedding planner if before putting on my dress I could squeeze in a ballet class—and I was only half kidding!

Nowadays, it's harder than ever to tune out the world around us and tune in to ourselves. We carry our social networks in our pockets, with everyone just a text or tweet away. That's why it's so essential to find ways to disconnect. Getting your body in motion is a great way to commune with your own thoughts and spirit.

Serotonin, a chemical that acts as a type of mental messenger, transmitting signals that impact everything from memory to mood, has been found to get a boost from exercise, and that means the more serotonin surging through our bodies, the stronger our feelings of tranquility.

When I am in ballet class, I get a feeling of serenity doing the steps that my muscles find familiar. Whatever activity you choose to do simply for pleasure, work on letting the distracting thoughts that pop up come and go, and try to stay mindful only of that moment.

Focus on your breathing as you jog. Revel in a bird's song as you stroll around your neighborhood. Feel the energy as your bike careens around a curve. Enjoy the silence that surrounds you when you dive underwater.

There are other activities that are less vigorous, more routine, but that may for you be just as calming. When you're in the kitchen, something as simple as chopping lettuce or seasoning vegetables can be soothing. Inhale the scents of the herbs, listen to the gentle rhythm of the knife nicking the cutting board. Don't think about the grocery run you have to make later, the test you have to take tomorrow, the disappointment you endured last week. Those tasks will still be there when you're done, or they will have already come and gone. Let's immerse ourselves in the here and now, moments set aside just for *you*.

Meditate to Contemplate

Meditation can quiet your mind and even help address some more serious challenges, such as anxiety and depression. There are different types of meditation, with some practitioners instructing that you sit a certain way or hold your hands in a particular position. By experimenting, you may discover that one variation feels more mellowing and beneficial than another. But the method I outline here is one that I think is simple enough for beginners to follow and is in keeping with my belief that becoming fit physically and emotionally should not require too many extra steps.

There are a few steps, however, that are crucial, like maintaining a strong posture. That's so you can forge a connection joining your mind, spirit, and body, a link as key to meditation as it will be to sculpting your ballerina body. So, to start:

- Sit up straight. If it helps, rest against a straight-backed chair or a wall.
- Shut your eyes and try to relax your shoulders and your arms so you are not coiled and tight. The goal is to allow your thoughts and emotions to flow, and a relaxed stance will help channel that energy.
- With your mouth closed, inhale through your nose to a count of four.
- Holding your breath, part your lips slightly. Then exhale through your mouth to a count of five.
- Repeat four or five times, or until you feel your body begin to relax into the rhythm.
- Thoughts will come up. You can't shut off your mind. But as those mental pictures emerge, try not to become caught up in them. Let them drift away, paying attention to your breathing to help pull you back.
- Try to meditate for at least five minutes, but fifteen to twenty minutes would be ideal. Try to sit in stillness for as long as you are able. It may be a bit difficult in the beginning, but the more you practice, the more natural it will feel.

SEEKING SANCTUARY

When we are still, we gain insight. We can connect with our inner compass, that subconscious voice that already knows the answers to our questions, the solution to that challenge that is keeping us awake at night. When we unclutter our minds, we create an opening to hear the internal messages that are often crowded out by the noise and stresses that surround us.

When you're writing in your journal, listening to music, engaging in meditation, or taking a brisk walk, you are able to retreat within yourself. To fully embrace those experiences, it's great to have a special place where you can burrow in and reflect.

That space is your designated go zone—the sanctuary you seek out to revive your spirit, and you can carve it out wherever you are. I can summon a sense of well-being at a table in the middle of a crowded dressing room. When I was a girl, growing up in San Pedro, I was soothed by the waves cresting and crashing at the beach. Think about where *you* find solitude, where you most feel in harmony with yourself.

It could be a corner of your family room. Stuff it with giant pillows or a comfortable chair. Tuck in a table and top it with candles. Or if you feel most alive when out in nature, spend time in your backyard or a local park. Even when it's winter, you can put on a warm jacket and enjoy communing with yourself while taking a walk.

Maybe you feel connected to the sacredness both inside and beyond yourself when you're in a house of worship. Or you might feel most relaxed and contemplative when you are in the bath. Turn the bathroom into your own personal spa. Fill it with salts and soaps, perfumes and potpourri, special scents that remind you that this is your personal time and it should be cherished.

In your sacred space, during your private moments, make sure the laptop is turned off and your smartphone is on silent. Or even better, leave your gadgets at home or stashed in another room—just for a little while. The only messages we are interested in during this precious time are the ones that arise from within.

Being mentally and emotionally grounded has helped me to weather criticism, injuries, and adversity. Creating moments and spaces that allow me to clear and quiet my mind has kept me centered and helped me to recover my confidence whenever I doubted myself. Finding the rituals and spaces that help you to stay balanced mentally, emotionally, and spiritually will keep you from being overwhelmed by life's many challenges and give you the subtle push you sometimes need to accomplish whatever you want. All the power you need is within *you*.

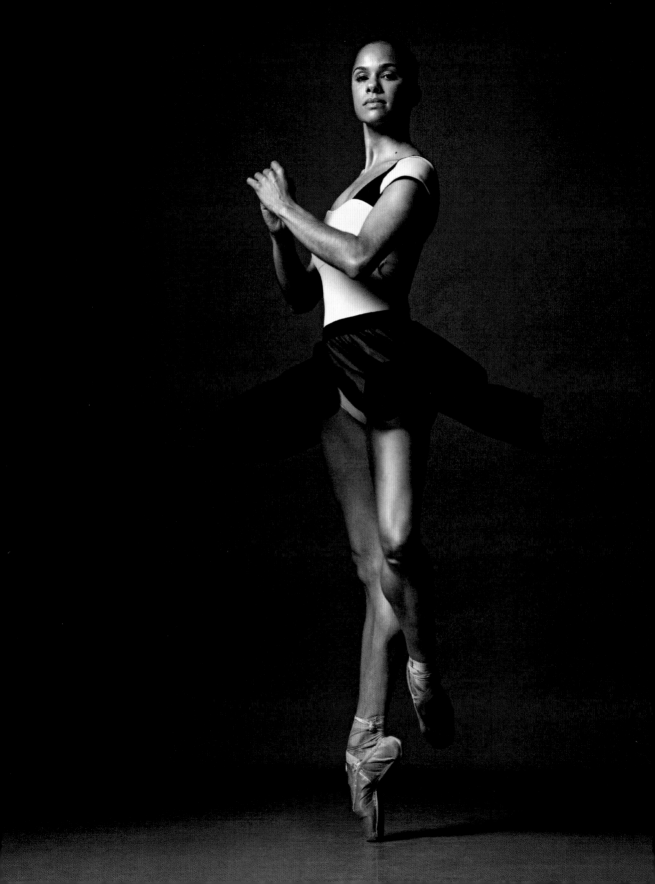

PART 2

Motion

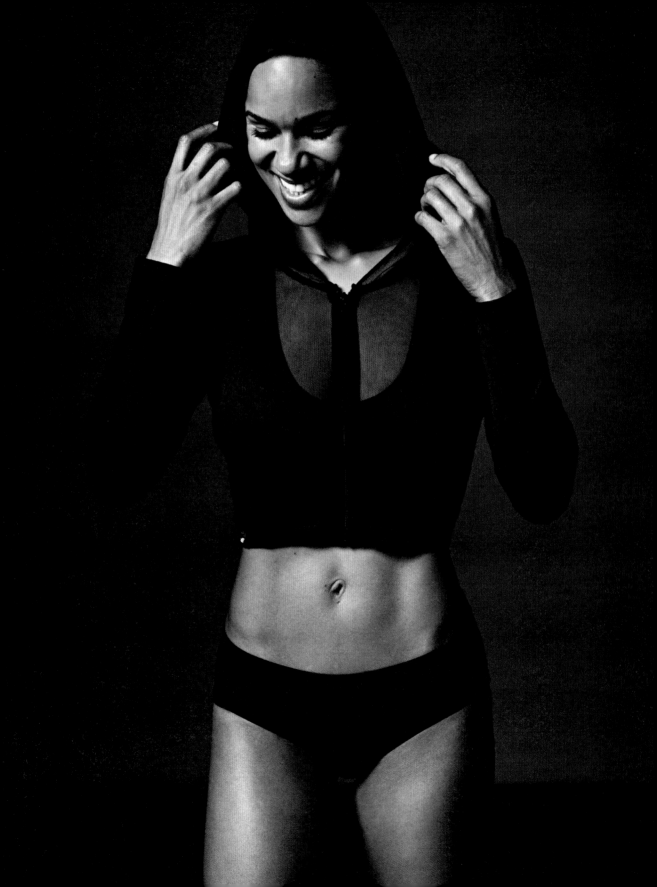

Chapter 4

IT'S NOT A WORKOUT— IT'S A WAY OF LIFE

Some of us think of a workout as a few hours a week confined to a gym, a chore that we have to endure and can't wait to get out of the way, or a short break where we can get our endorphins surging before heading back to the more mundane tasks filling our afternoon.

But fitness shouldn't be thought of as just an aerobic intermission, an isolated and intermittent part of our daily routines. Working out, so essential to our mental and physical well-being, can and should be woven through every part of our lives. After all, exercising is a microcosm of life: to make the most of both, you need the same elements—discipline, strength, a sense of connection, and, perhaps most important, balance.

Our health is on the line in the United States. More than a third of adults were obese at the start of this decade, and 17 percent of children and teenagers were also considered extremely overweight. That can be dangerous, raising the chance for so many maladies, including type 2 diabetes and high blood pressure. We want to take as many steps as we can to prevent illness and overcome health challenges that we may be facing, and fitness—along with proper nutrition—is a key part of the solution.

You don't have to wait until you get off work or out of school to head to the nearest spin class. We can incorporate extra movements into our everyday activities, toning our calves as we stand at the bus stop, strengthening our core and lengthening our arm muscles while sitting at our desks, and giving our limbs a good energizing stretch before we even get out of bed. And at all times, in whatever position, we can and should practice strong posture.

STANDING TALL

I don't recall if I always had good posture, but I think I always had an awareness of my body. Maybe because I was so self-conscious as a child, my voice and sense of self often shrunken inside, I felt a need to physically stand tall, whether I was doing my job as a middle school hall monitor or directing my peers as captain of the drill team. I guess I understood even then, before I found ballet, that a regal pose displayed confidence whether or not I actually felt it. And if your body projected it, eventually your mind would believe it.

Good posture—your back erect, your shoulders even and relaxed, your face peering straight ahead—magnifies your presence. It gives you poise, a bearing, that lets bystanders in every class you sit in, on every street you walk down, in every room you enter, know that, *yes*, you have arrived.

Do you remember how seeing is believing? How when we visualize our goals, chronicle our dreams, etch our future on a vision board, we can help spin our desires into reality? *Feeling* is believing as well. When we stand tall, we feel powerful, and that energy can propel us forward in any endeavor we want to take on.

Posture, you see, is really *all* about energy. That is something that we dancers quickly come to understand. We cannot dance fully and freely if our bodies aren't held in a way that allows our breath and energy to circulate, unimpeded, from head to toe. That is what gives us our power and ignites the invisible spark that connects ourselves, our fellow dancers, and the audience and that can help our performances transcend technical precision and soar to a place that is ethereal and magical.

We learn as dancers that our stance encompasses more than our upper backs and shoulders, and standing tall does more than just strengthen our core. We must take possession, take control, of our entire bodies to manifest as much fluidity, strength, and grace as possible.

Strong posture is perhaps the first and most basic step toward honing your ballerina body. When your stance is solid, it keeps you conscious of your physical self, reminding you constantly of how vital your body is and how important it is to do all you can to nurture and strengthen it.

Posture is also essential to your workout, creating a channel of energy that flows freely from your mind, through your core, and down to your toes. That sparks both a physical and a mental connection that will help you power through your exercises.

Many of our bodies have curled into a slight slouch that comes from sitting at desks much of the day, or hunching over our cell phones. But just the way strong posture becomes programmed into the muscles and skeletal structure of professional dancers, practicing an elegant stance can similarly fire up your muscle memory, becoming a form that your body slips into naturally. You can retrain your muscles to push up against gravity, maintaining a steady connection between your mind and your core, which will make your workout ever-more effective.

Stretches to Help with Posture

1. When you find yourself slouching, stand, clasp your hands behind you, and then stretch them down and away from your body. While doing this, you may find that your head goes slightly forward or back. This is fine. Try the stretch both ways: Let your head fall forward as you stretch your arms behind you. Then try it allowing your head to go back, looking up. Do not stay in this position longer than feels comfortable; a few seconds is enough. Release and come back to a neutral stance. Repeat in the direction—head forward or head backward—that feels the most helpful, as that is what your body needs at the time. For some, both directions relieve tensions.

2. Whenever you have a towel (which is probably at least twice a day) or a long belt in your hands, hold it so there's enough space between your hands for you to bring it over your head without bending your elbows. Bring it behind you and back again, again without bending your elbows or losing the symmetry in your shoulders. Do this two or three times in a row, keeping a slow tempo.

So many benefits flow from good posture and holding your core strong when you stand and walk. Good posture opens up your diaphragm, helping you to breathe better, and that in turn can help you to remain calm and in the moment—another mind-body link that can keep you grounded, literally and mentally, throughout your day.

Standing erect can boost your health as well. It aids good digestion and it can ward off arthritis by keeping the surface of your joints intact. It relieves pressure on the spine and helps to ensure that your muscles aren't being overtaxed, because the surrounding bones and joints are kept in the proper position. In fact, the strong physical alignment that is a hallmark of dance is one of the reasons it attracts many people suffering from scoliosis, an excessive curvature of the spine.

So, when you're practicing strong posture, remember all that you are accomplishing. You are clearing a path for the energy that flows through you from head to toe. You may be fortifying yourself against future injury and safeguarding your muscles and joints. And all the while, you'll look fierce, confident, and powerful.

EXERCISE TO GO

With fitness being so integral to health, the ideal way to get all the activity our minds and bodies need is to integrate movement into all aspects of our lives. Not only does that mean being able to perform your Ballerina Body routines wherever you are, be it a dorm room, your house, or a hotel, but it also means being able to hone your physique when you are at work, at play, or shuttling in between.

- Climb the stairs whenever possible.
- Park the car far from the store and walk briskly there and back.
- Toss a Frisbee at the park.
- Jog through the waves during a day at the beach.

We can also start incorporating some of our Ballerina Body moves into our everyday routines to start sculpting our bodies, or at least to begin warming them up in preparation for our full-on exercise routine. Many of these "to-go" exercises are basically simplified versions of what we'll do in Chapter 5.

Eye-Opener

You can start seconds after you open your eyes, first thing in the morning, while lying in bed. When you are just shaking off sleep, you don't want to move too abruptly, throwing off the covers and leaping to your feet. But there's a move that you can do to gently awaken your body, preparing it for all the physical activity—including your official workout—you will engage in throughout the rest of the day. (This is a variation of the Tension Release exercise in Chapter 5, page 44.)

a. While lying in bed, either on your back or on your side, tighten yourself into a ball. Squeeze as tightly as you can.

b. Then, holding that shape, raise your shoulders against the base of your skull at the back of your head, known as the occipital ridge. Hold for five seconds, then release. Repeat.

c. Next, release the tension in your muscles, freely stretching all parts of your body— arms, legs, torso—in all directions. You should feel the tension fade away.

d. Linger for a few moments, then gently swing your legs over the edge of the bed, plant your feet on the ground, and slowly stand and begin your day.

Posting

If you have a stationary chair—one that isn't rolling around on wheels—this is an exercise you can do while sitting at your desk or watching television. It will foster good posture and give your hamstrings and sitz bones a workout whose impact you'll notice when you are able to walk farther, dance longer, and engage in other sports with more vigor. (We will repeat this exercise in Chapter 5, page 45.)

a. Sit with your feet parallel to each other and planted on the floor. They should be in line with your hips. Your hands may rest, palms down, on the thighs, with arms relaxed, while you maintain good posture.

b. Gently press the soles of your feet, even if you're wearing shoes, firmly against the ground.

c. Then, gently squeeze the hamstrings in the backs of your thighs. (Do not purposely squeeze the buttocks. The impetus should come from using the hamstrings. The buttocks will be affected, without tucking under, when the stretch is done properly.)

d. Again, do not tuck under your backside while doing this! We'll talk more about this later, but tucking under can bulk up your thigh muscles rather than contouring and elongating them.

e. The squeeze should hike you up on the chair. This is the same technique used when riding a trotting horse, but it is not necessary to ride horses to utilize the same muscles, the hamstrings, at the backs of the thighs. The identified and strengthened hamstrings will help to hold you upright, encouraging good posture.

f. Do repeatedly, alternately squeezing and releasing, for about a minute. Then start again. Exhale normally as you squeeze. Inhale as you release. There is no need to exaggerate your breath. When this becomes easy to do, you may squeeze for two breaths/release the hold on the last inhale, then three breaths; but always breathe without stress.

g. Do as many repetitions as you wish, but try to do this move at least three times.

Torso Turn

This is a great way to target your core abdominal muscles, engaging them and giving them a good stretch. It also gives you a break if you're staring at a computer or doing other work. It's a way to take a few moments to focus on *you*. (This is an exercise that we will repeat in Chapter 5, page 46.)

a. Start as if you were doing the Posting exercise: feet parallel and planted on the floor.

b. With your feet flat on the floor, your hips facing forward, your back straight, and your shoulder blades down, do the Posting lift.

c. Then turn the upper part of your torso to the right, draping your right arm over the back of your seat, and gently stretch your upper body toward the floor while keeping your hips facing forward, in line with your knees and toes.

d. Bring your arm back gently to your side, and turn your torso back to the center.

e. Repeat the same motions on your left side.

f. Try to do at least five stretches on each side, but do as many as you can for as long as you can.

Pulse

This is a way to begin chiseling your ballerina calves while you're waiting for the bus, washing dishes, folding laundry, or standing in line at the movies or the bookstore. It can be done with or without shoes, but if you are wearing shoes, make sure they are flat, without a heel.

Grab hold of something firm—the edge of a sink, the washing machine, or even a heavy table will do. Then:

a. Rise onto the balls of your feet.

b. Pulse your feet up and down without touching your heels to the ground for ten seconds. This can also be done with one foot in front of the other, starting a calf stretch. Keep your legs parallel, toes facing forward. With your front leg bent, and your weight on it, put the other foot back and keep the back leg straight, and about twelve inches behind the hip on that side. Begin pulsing the heel of your back leg up and down, about two or three inches, to lengthen and stretch out tight calves and Achilles tendons. The weight should be kept over the front leg and foot during this exercise. Then switch your legs' positions and repeat the exercise.

c. Repeat for as long as you can, but try to increase your number of reps over time.

d. Lower your heels to the ground.

Note: You can also do the Pulse by standing still on the balls of your feet for a count of three, then lowering your heels to the floor. Again, feel free to hold on to a chair, rail, or other stable surface, though the more you work out, the better your balance is sure to become.

Head, Neck, and Shoulder Roll

This is a way to get your body moving from the shoulders up. You can do it pretty much anywhere, anytime, but think about it in the morning, perhaps after you brush your teeth or while you're checking your email, and anytime you need a quick stress reliever during your day. (This is a simpler version of the Head, Neck, and Shoulder Roll we will do in Chapter 5, page 44.)

a. Throughout this stretch, keep your torso, shoulders, and arms relaxed, not tight. Let your arms sway freely.

b. Hold your head high. Tilt it gently forward, only as far as it will go without straining. Return your head to center after it reaches the forward limit, then gently lean your head back, again returning it upright after it has gone as far back as is comfortably possible. Repeat three times.

c. Next, turn your head to the right, bring it back to the center, and then turn it to the left. Repeat three times on each side.

d. Then face forward.

e. Tilt your head to bring your right ear toward your right shoulder. When it can go no farther, bring the head upright and tilt the left ear toward the left shoulder, returning it to center. Repeat three times.

f. Again, bring your head easily forward, then softly circle your head to one side, then circle your head back toward your other shoulder, then continue forward. Repeat two or three times.

g. Next, lift your shoulders and touch the base of your skull to your right shoulder, and then roll your head back and to your left, gently massaging the muscles along the base of your skull. Repeat to suit your needs. (If at any point you encounter tension, make small movements up and down against the tightness.)

READY, SET, GO

Motion isn't an aside to our daily lives. It's essential to maintaining our health and stamina, flooding our bodies with the feel-good chemicals that give us peace, and enabling us to do all that matters most to us—studying, cultivating our careers, spending quality time with friends and family, and pursuing the activities and interests that give us joy.

Now that you know a few everyday moves that you can do while lying in bed, sitting in your office or classroom, or standing in line, it's time to get into the official moves that will help sculpt your ballerina body. Let's go!

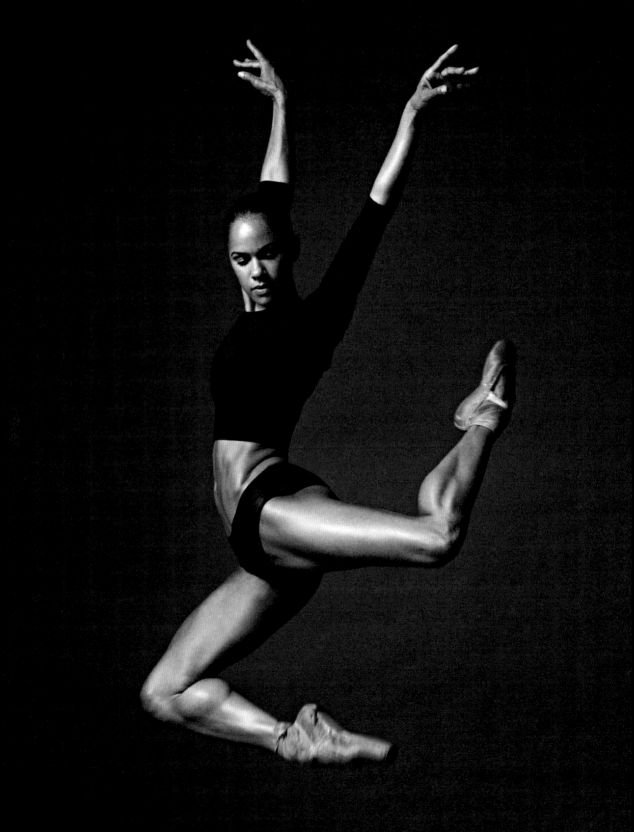

Chapter 5

BALLERINA MOVES

My body has always moved with ease. Though that's changed a bit with age, my limbs have been loose and flexible for as long as I can remember. We all have our similarities as well as our unique qualities. Some people wake up ready to move, like I do, while others find that they are stiff in one part of their body or another when they first open their eyes.

Those differences are true even among professional dancers. Every dancer has a way of preparing for class or exercise that is uniquely beneficial to her or him. For instance, I tend to tire with too much warm-up preparation or repetition of exercises, while some of my peers need the extra reps to feel completely ready to go.

I think that most dancers prepare for their dancing lives with every move they make, in every moment of the day. And I believe that even if you are not aiming for a professional dance career and simply want to look and feel your best, you can achieve those results by being dedicated physically and emotionally and maintaining a positive spirit.

Let's begin with the moment we open our eyes after a night's sleep and let our eyes adjust to the light. In that same way, our bodies should be prepared before jumping out of bed, landing all our weight on the feet and ankles. A cat never wakes up, jumps up, and runs across the room. Instead, cats tend to enjoy a good stretch before darting off. Why not take inspiration from nature? Here are a few exercises to get you going.

1. Tension Release

These moves are a great way for anyone to start the morning, though I think every dancer begins the day with some form of these tension releasers. (This is a variation of the Eye-Opener exercise in Chapter 4, page 37.)

    a. While still in bed, curl your body into a tight ball—tighter and tighter. Then let all the tightness go. Notice the tension slipping away, freeing the body.

    b. Next, stretch your body freely in every direction that feels good, all at once. Try to imagine opening all of your joints and stretching your muscles. Again, let all the tension go.

2. Head, Neck, and Shoulder Roll

Get your head, neck, shoulders, and arms moving freely once you're up and out of bed. Try improvising movement, but if you need some suggestions for how to begin relaxing and energizing your muscles and joints to start your day, here are some basic moves that you can do to release any tension in your neck and shoulders before challenging your body with more vigorous exercises or simply going about your usual activities. (This is a variation of the exercise we did in Chapter 4, page 40.)

    a. First lift your chin slightly, then let your head gradually fall forward. Lift your head upright again, then repeat, slowly, two or three times. We lift the chin up before moving the head forward or backward to create space in the spine. That will prevent pinching in the spine and shoulders.

    b. Slowly turn your head from side to side, two or three times to each side. Then face forward again.

    c. Now tilt your head to the right to move your right ear toward your right shoulder. Bring your head upright again, then tilt your head so your left ear moves toward your left shoulder. Repeat this two or three times to each side. Gently circle your head to one side, then circle it in the other direction. Take your time.

    d. Lift your shoulders and lean the base of the back of your skull (the occipital ridge) toward your shoulders, alternately moving your head to the left and right to massage the muscles at the back of your neck and the base of your skull against your shoulders. If at any point you encounter tension, make small movements up and down against the tightness. These movements should be free, led by the feelings you get as you relieve tension.

e. Release your shoulders.

f. Gently sway. Move your torso and your arms freely.

Even if you think you don't have time, these are exercises you can do as you go through your morning rituals, as you prepare breakfast, check email, or wash your hands or the dishes. As I said before, this stretching regimen can also be achieved naturally, fluidly, without choreography. Yes, I'm a dancer and I'm used to following a certain set of steps, but feel free to create your own routine and pattern for these movements, one that is right for you and for how your body is feeling on a given day.

3. Feet

This exercise can be done before getting out of bed, or while you're sitting at the breakfast table or on the train.

a. Flex your toes and ankles, then point your ankles and toes, in that order, so that you're not starting with your toes from a flexed foot, or starting with your ankles from a pointed foot.

b. Add slow circles, rotating your feet and ankles in both directions. Make easy circles, not the biggest circles you can make.

4. Posting

This has become one of my favorite exercises. (We also did this in Chapter 4, page 37.) When you get into your groove and really activate the right muscles, you feel like you can jump from any position, or even fly. Ha!

Both Posting and the Torso Turn (following) can be done at any time of day. A few repetitions at a time can be enough. Never force this or any other movements or exercises.

This exercise is like posting to the trot on a horse (the up-and-down motion riders use in rhythm with a horse's trot), but you do it while sitting in a firm, stable chair.

a. Sit with your feet well planted on the floor, parallel, about hip distance from each other. The hands may rest, palms down, on the thighs, with arms relaxed, while you maintain good posture.

b. Gently press the soles of your feet (even inside shoes) firmly against the floor.

c. Find what my floor barre instructor, Marjorie Liebert, likes to call the bookends (the sides of the body running from your armpits to the outside of your heels). Feel energy from the bookends evenly pulling toward each other. Imagine that you're holding the body as bookends supporting a row of books. If this is too large an area to identify, first begin with the sides of the pelvis and upper thighs. The legs and inner thighs (adductors) should remain parallel and symmetrical. We strive for symmetry, as much as possible. This will encourage good posture as well.

d. Once you're in this position, it is easier to squeeze the hamstrings gently toward each other and release, repeatedly, without igniting the tuck-under muscles (gluteus maximus), as we do not want to tuck under. The squeeze should bring you up on the chair and release you down as you let go, like posting on a horse.

Isolating these muscles can serve you well for pretty much everything, whether you're dancing, playing a sport, walking, or simply sitting. It directs energy to the hamstrings, which radiates to the rest of the body, including lifting the glutes.

5. Torso Turn

This is an exercise we also did in Chapter 4, page 38.

a. In the same position we started Posting in—feet planted on the floor, hips facing front, posture erect, shoulder blades down, using the Posting lift to start—turn your upper torso to the left side.

b. Drape your left arm over the back of the chair and gently stretch, turning left at the waist while keeping the hips, knees, and feet facing front. Let the arm come back to your side and return your torso to center.

c. Repeat on the other side.

FLOOR EXERCISES

Now we can get to our floor work. The floor will be the base for our initial exercises, helping to build an understanding of the movements you will eventually do standing up. While you are lying down, your muscles will gain the memory, coordination, and strength that will enable you to do the standing exercises more safely.

These exercises are a basic way to do the floor work suitable for most beginners. When comfortable with the basic steps, you can make the exercises more advanced by adding head movements, arm movements, or both to the leg movements described. More complex choreography can be substituted for some of the exercises. And if you like to move to music—which can give you an extra burst of energy, making exercise more fun—you can alternate the rhythms of certain exercises by changing the sound track. Again, this is a basic plan. Many more exercises can be added or substituted.

However, please remember with these and all our other movements, never to force yourself to the point that it hurts! And here's another important rule: For all floor work done on the back, when both legs are bent or both legs are in the air, the lower back must hug the floor to prevent back problems. While you're lying on your back and lengthening your legs, your lower back is released from the floor, while as many ribs in your back as comfortably possible remain on the ground. In other words, do not arch your back!

Also, to sit up from a lying position on your back, bend your legs at the knees until the soles of your feet rest on the floor. Then sit up as you stretch your legs along the floor.

Here's a more advanced approach to sitting up without having to bend the knees, then straighten them. But do not try this too early in your workout journey, as sitting and lying down this way is more difficult than any of the exercises.

a. Hold your back strong without disrupting or bending anywhere but at the hip.

b. Hold your arms out at your sides on the floor, hands a bit above your shoulders, with your palms facing down.

c. Keep your knees straight as you use your arms and the backs of your legs to press into the floor, with your energy going through the floor and out of your feet.

d. As you lift your chest up toward the ceiling, propelling your torso to come off the floor and forward to sitting, try not to release at the rib cage or the waist (no arching or collapsing the spine). The same is done in reverse as you lie down.

6. Hip Opener

We want to create the optimum space in the joints, allowing you to move freely. This exercise can be done while lying on your stomach and again while lying on your back.

a. Lie on your stomach, head turned to the right, left cheek on the floor. Your legs should be extended, and relaxed; your arms bent at a ninety-degree angle with your palms facing down. With your foot relaxed and on the floor, slide your right leg along the floor, with your knee bent toward your right elbow, without forcing. Be comfortable, as this is movement therapy, not exercise. Keeping your foot re-laxed, slide your right leg back toward your left leg until it's back at the starting position.

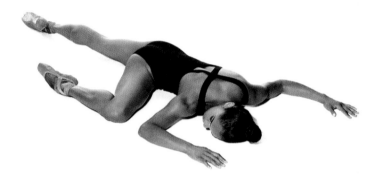

b. Do not hold the rest of your body rigid; instead, allow your core and your stationary leg to freely let go of their positions. Repeat the movement, and on the third rep-etition of bringing your knee toward your elbow, lift your foot and lower leg, turning them in and pulling your knee toward your standing leg. (The non-moving leg is called the standing leg, even when you're lying on the floor. The moving leg is called the working leg.)

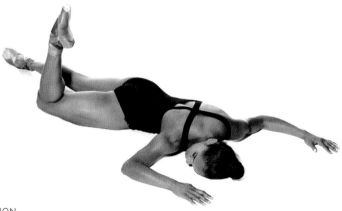

c. Repeat this step once, your knee out, turning your foot up to the ceiling and then dragging your knee in toward the standing leg. Then return your leg to lengthen it next to the standing leg.

d. Turn your head and repeat the whole combination with the other leg.

e. Repeat the entire exercise, this time lying on your back. Remember, don't force it. This is a good warm-up exercise, but it can also be used for cooldown or anytime you're feeling out of sorts or in need of freedom through the back, pelvis, or both.

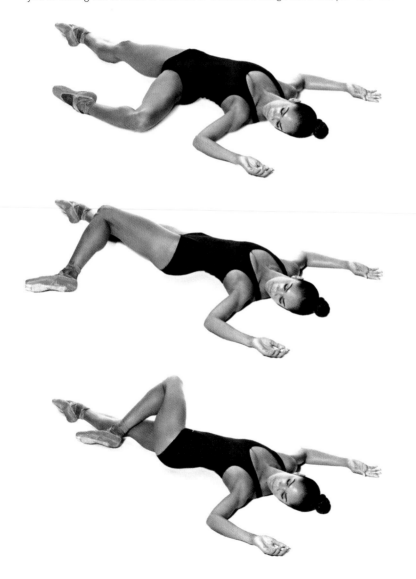

7. X, I, T, G

This series of exercises opens channels of energy in the body. It can be done at any time, whenever you want to work the kinks out, as long as you have enough space to lie down. If you have time to do only X and I, or T, or T and G, that too can be beneficial.

X

a. Lie on your back with your legs and arms open on the floor, like a human X. Without taking any of your limbs off the floor, reach one arm up over your head while reaching down with the opposite leg. Release.

b. Repeat with the other diagonal stretch of arm and leg.

c. Do this three or four times on each side.

I

a. Now bring your arms closer together, right above your head. Bring your legs closer together, too, without force—you are looking for them to stay as close as they can stay on their own.

b. This time, extend your right arm and right leg away from each other in opposite directions. Then do the same on the other side, repeating three or four times on each side.

T

a. Still lying on your back, bend your legs, putting the soles of your feet on the floor so that your lower back hugs the floor.

b. Place your arms out to your sides, palms facing up, just below your shoulders.

c. Now, release your lower back, rolling onto the tip of your tailbone. (When the lower back arches, we find ourselves naturally rolling to the tip of the tailbone.) Then push your lower back to the floor again; feel your breath filling the lower back, while feeling your lower back muscles hugging the floor, as you stretch your arms to the sides along the floor with shoulders relaxed.

d. Release and repeat three or four times.

a. From the T position, with your lower back feeling the floor, bring your legs up into the air, one at a time, putting your right hand on your right leg just below your kneecap, and your left hand on your left leg.

b. At the same time, while exhaling, curl your upper back off the floor around your lower abs, with your shoulder blades pointing down in the direction of your waist.

c. While inhaling, release and roll down.

d. Press your shins into your hands again, holding your breath briefly.

e. Curl up around your lower abs, exhaling. Inhale as you roll down.

f. Repeat this whole sequence, exhaling as you curl up and inhaling as you release down, as many times as you like.

This is excellent and safe work for strengthening the lower abs and the lower back.

8. Back Stretch

Marjorie Liebert, who has instructed me in floor barre, has dubbed this exercise my specialty. I think it's because it makes me feel like I am dancing while lying on my back, especially when I was injured with my tibia stress fractures. I felt so free when doing this.

There are a number of variations of this warm-up stretch, but this is a good one, generally suitable for most people, from beginners to advanced students who've had no injury or surgery to make it too difficult. You can do this stretch as a warm-up movement and also to cool down. This can also be done, gently, anytime your back is feeling tight or achy.

a. Lie on your back with your legs bent, the soles of your feet on the floor, and your legs hip distance apart. Make sure your lower back is firmly supported by the floor.

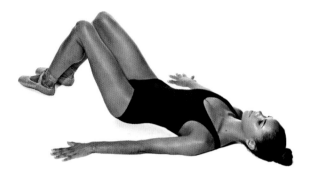

b. Stretch your arms to the sides, just below shoulder height, palms down. Your arms help to balance your core by hugging the floor as your legs move.

c. Allow your knees to lead your legs to fall in one direction while your head drops to the other side as you exhale.

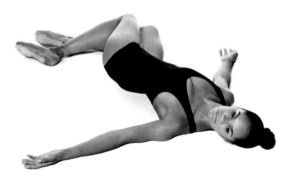

d. Return your legs and head to center, inhaling. Do the same movement to the other side. Return to the center.

9. Plié

"Plié" means "fold" or "bend" in French. This is the first exercise we dancers do every day in ballet class to warm up. And it's just as beneficial when you do it on the floor!

Pliés warm up the joints and get the muscle groups to work together, as well as lining up the spine for good posture. Start with four sets of pliés with the legs parallel, and four sets with the legs turned out; one set with flexed feet and one set with pointed feet—and always flex toes then ankles and point ankles then toes.

In every exercise we do, when you are flexing your feet, try to envision sending energy away from your body, through the soles of your feet.

You will do this exercise on your back and on your stomach.

a. Begin by lying on your back with your legs parallel, big toe joints touching each other. With your feet pointed, bend (plié) your legs simultaneously until your lower back touches the floor—without tucking, pinching the muscles of the buttocks and sending the tailbone between the legs. (This move can also be done with your feet flexed, if pointed is too difficult to maintain.) Try not to tense or grip the joints in your ankles, which must remain supple and free.

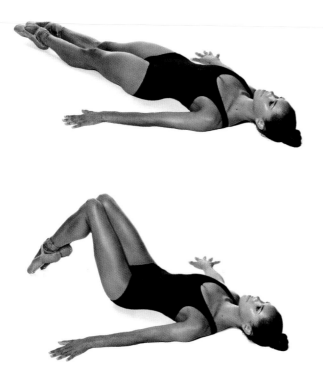

b. Next, lengthen your legs, gently releasing your back from the floor, using the floor to guide the movement. With your legs elongated along the floor, flex your toes and then your ankles, and point your ankles, then your toes. (Reverse this sequence when starting with your feet flexed.) With your feet flexed, bend your legs until your lower back touches the floor.

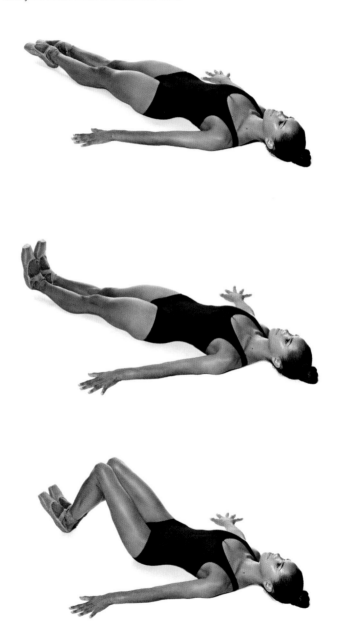

c. Repeat the pliés four times in the turned-out position (knees pointed toward the walls on either side), heels lifted off the floor if possible; if not possible, they may relax on the floor until you are able to lift them with either pointed or flexed feet. Remember, when both knees are bent, at the top of the plié, or both legs are in the air, the lower spine touches the floor. Two pliés followed by two point/flex equals one repetition. Beginning with your heels together and your feet pointed, bend your knees until your toes meet, your heels separate, and your lower back finds the support of the floor. Then reverse the sequence, toes together until your heels meet as your legs straighten to first position (heels touching, feet either pointed— more advanced—or flexed), during which your lower back comfortably releases from the floor. Lengthen your legs until they are straight.

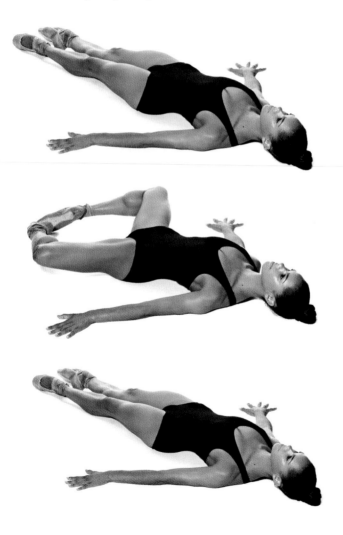

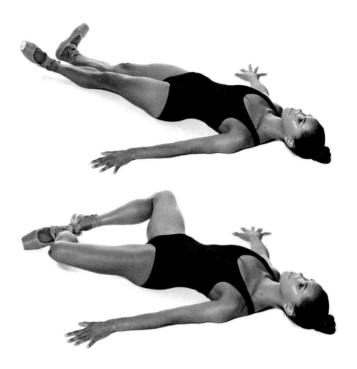

d. Repeat this exercise while lying on your stomach. To start, place one hand on top of the other and place your forehead on the top hand. When you are feeling confident and strong, you can place your arms at your sides, at right angles, with your hands and elbows carrying equal weight and in line with each other.

e. Now, lying on your stomach, repeat the pliés four times in the parallel position, keeping your legs stretched and connected to your core as you flex and point. Next do four sets of pliés in the turned-out position (en dehors). If you begin with your feet flexed, your heels will stay together as you plié and straighten your legs. When you are in first position, stretch your ankles, then your toes, creating properly pointed feet; follow with flexing your toes, then your ankles, doing the point and flex twice.

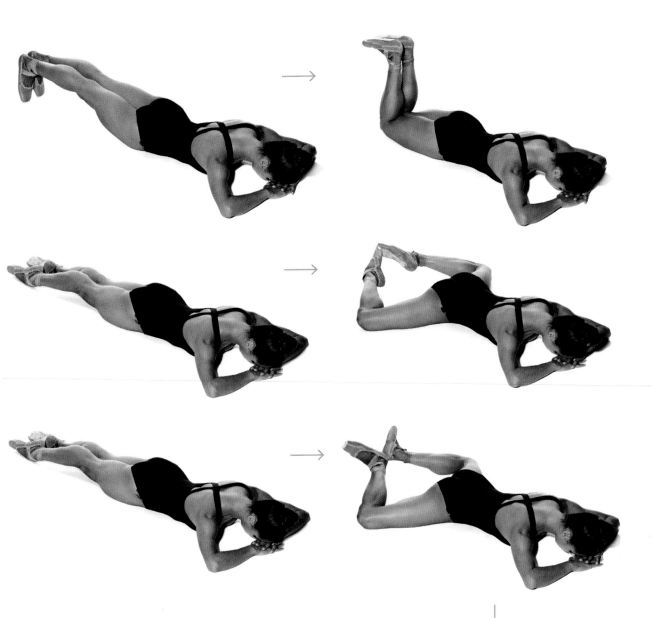

f. Do the same exercise: two pliés and two flexes and points of the feet. Do not arch your back while you are working through your pliés and flexes and points. Hold your core stable, moving only your legs.

10. Butterfly

This is a basic stretch you learn at a very young age in ballet. It's a good and easy one to start to gain more turnout in your hips. You'll get freedom in your hip sockets and strength and stability through your back and limbs.

You will do this on your back and your stomach, with flexed and pointed feet.

a. To start, lie on your back with your legs together, bent, and your arms down by your sides, palms facing down. Begin with flexed feet. (When you feel ready and confident, you can start with pointed feet.)

b. Keeping your lower back firmly planted on the floor, open your knees outward to the sides, as far as they will go without releasing your lower back from the floor, creating the butterfly position. Then close your knees together.

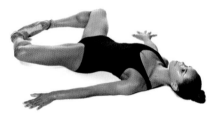

c. Repeat the opening of your knees, then bring the knees up about one-eighth of the way and immediately let them fall open to the limit determined by the lower back hugging the floor, while directing the knees toward the side walls, without releasing the stability through your back and your center. When your back remains on the floor, energy is able to travel through your back and arms, as well as your legs. The release and second opening of the knees occurs when your legs can go no farther without disturbing your posture.

d. Repeat this exercise (opening your knees, closing them about one-eighth of the way, and releasing again) two more times so you've done three full openings of your turnout, with the lower back remaining on the floor. Then open, close, and open your knees.

e. If you began with flexed feet, repeat with pointed feet, when you are able.

f. Lengthen your legs to the floor, comfortably turned out (heels together, toes apart).

g. With your arms pressing the floor and your lower back returning to the floor, hold your legs in first position (heels together, toes apart and pointed) and lift them into the air until they are at a ninety-degree angle with your hips (making an L shape with your body and legs), bending your legs until the feet are on the floor. Then stretch the lower legs, straight up, toes pointed toward the ceiling.

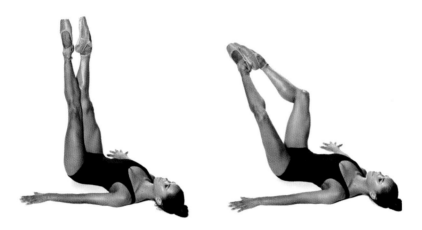

h. As you bend your knees—plié—your toes will touch the floor, still turned out.

i. Repeat this sequence from turned out to parallel, always mindful that your spine's relationship to the floor is a priority. You will bring your legs up to ninety degrees parallel, this time.

j. Repeat the Butterfly on your stomach, lengthening your legs until your feet touch the floor instead of ninety degrees, then lengthening the legs, after the butterfly (in and out) movements. Again, your core being well placed determines the limit of the opening of your legs.

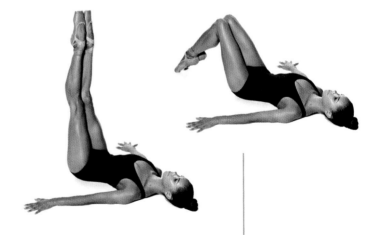

11. Plié en Dehors with Extension

With this exercise, your warm-up continues with the addition of the back of your legs (hamstrings) and your inner thighs (adductors). Do this exercise on your back and then on your stomach. As a beginner, you should begin with flexed feet, lying on your back. Later, when you are feeling more comfortable with the exercise, begin with pointed feet while lying on your back.

a. Plié in the turned-out position (en dehors), and then straighten your legs outward to the sides in an open V, without forcing your legs too wide as you lengthen them. In this position, flex and point your feet, or point and flex your feet. If you're a beginner, start with flexed feet.

b. Next, plié en dehors, with your lower back touching the floor, and both legs bent in the turned-out position.

c. Now lengthen your legs to first position (heels together, toes apart), releasing your lower back as you stretch your knees.

d. Repeat four times on your back and four times on your stomach.

12. Walk

The leg lifts and pulsing in the walk are great for alignment, warming up the hip flexors, and strengthening the abs, glutes, and posture.

While doing the walks, use your arms on the floor by your sides to support your back. Your arms will help to hold the sides of your body from the armpits to the outer anklebones (bookends), centering the core and preventing you from sitting into your hips and your outer legs.

a. Lying on your back with your knees bent in parallel (lower back hugging the floor, as is the rule) and feet fully on the floor, lift one leg, still in the bent position as though you are walking, with a relaxed foot (not flexed or pointed) two inches off the floor, then put it down.

b. Repeat with the other leg.

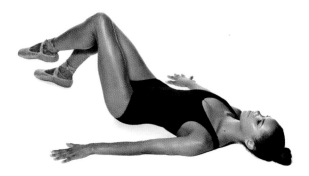

c. Continue the walks three more times, lengthening your leg into the air on the fifth
lift, at which time you may flex or point.

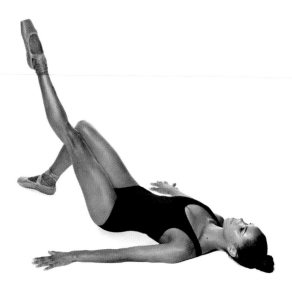

d. Pulse the stretched leg up and down, just an inch or two, several times. Use your
arms, palms down, to stabilize your core.

e. Put the lifted foot on the floor and repeat, beginning with the other leg.

13. Dégagé

"Dégagé" means "disengaged." When preparing for dégagés in particular, but whenever you're lying on the floor, you should feel like you are standing or jumping—not lying on the sand at the beach!

This exercise is good for length, strength, and alignment. Be sure to press the parts of your back and body that are touching the surface of the floor to the floor, allowing your working leg to float up, initiating the movement with your inner thighs and the backs of the legs rather than the top of your thighs (quadriceps).

a. Begin lying on your back with your feet in first position (heels together and toes apart, feet pointed).

b. Place your arms at your sides with your palms facing down; you can vary the positioning of your arms depending on what makes you comfortable, as long as your arms don't go above your shoulders.

c. Keep your legs elongated, straight on the floor.

d. Use your palms and arms by pressing them to the floor. This will help to strengthen your core and align the spine.

e. Lift one leg two or three inches from the floor, with your toes still pointed out, by pressing the standing leg (again, whether you're standing or lying on the floor, the standing leg is the one that is not moving; it helps to maintain balance), your arms, and your head into the floor. This will help you to lift the working leg while maintaining stability throughout your body. Do four dégagés with one leg front, then switch legs and do four with the other leg front.

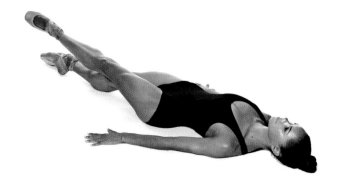

f. Now do four dégagés to each side. For these, your working leg stays on the floor, brushing along the floor as it extends to the side. Do not disturb the balance of the pelvis or the back as you move the working leg.

14. Seaweed

This exercise is great for freeing and lengthening the spine and for centering and strengthening the core.

a. Begin lying on your back, your legs together and parallel and your feet pointed.

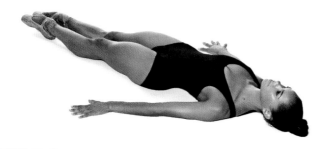

b. Bend your legs slowly, bringing them off the floor, still bent, and lifting your feet off the floor as well, while your back hugs the ground.

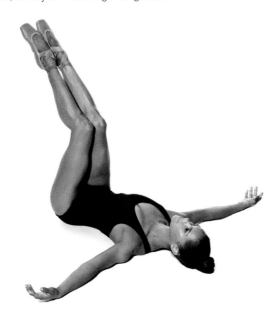

c. Keeping your lower back on the floor and your shoulder blades drawn toward your waist, curl your upper back off the floor, around your lower abs. Your arms should act like seaweed being moved by the motion of the tides, around and behind your lifted legs.

d. Float your upper back and arms down to the floor, legs still bent, body still energized.

e. Repeat four times, bringing your legs gently toward your head as your core and upper body lift, igniting the lower abdominal muscles.

f. After the last time, hold one hand or wrist (depending on the length of your arms) with the other, behind your thighs.

g. Lengthen your legs straight into the air, pressing the backs of your legs into your arms.

h. Propel your legs to the floor, arms still around them, until you get close to the floor. Then open your arms to the sides and move them forward toward your feet, over your head.

i. Your upper back should bend forward over your legs as you transition from lying to sitting, with the backs of your hands on the floor to help stabilize and keep the backs of your legs on the floor.

j. Roll down through your spine until your back is on the floor and you are in the starting position, with your shoulders relaxed. Repeat two to four times.

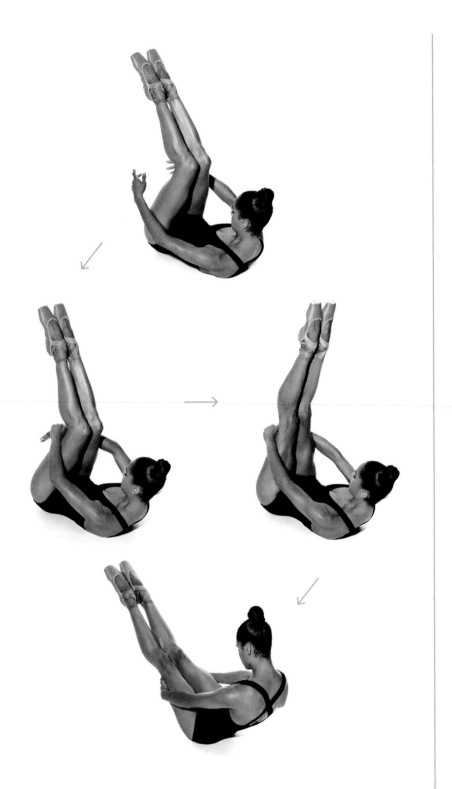

15. Rond de Jambe

"Rond de jambe" refers to the working leg making a circle around the standing leg. This exercise will help free the hip sockets and legs from the joints.

a. Start by lying on your back, your knees bent, both feet on the floor.

b. Lift one leg up, lengthening it toward the ceiling, with a pointed foot, until it's at a ninety-degree angle to the floor. Turn it out. Keep your other leg bent, with your foot on the floor.

c. With the extended leg, make four small circles to the outside (en dehors), then four small circles to the inside (en dedans).

d. Then make bigger, but still controlled, circles, again four en dehors and four en dedans. Return the working leg to the floor, turned parallel, after the fourth repetition, and perform the same exercise with the other leg.

e. After repeating the sequence with the other leg, return to the starting position of two bent knees, both feet on the floor. Now lengthen your legs as you sit up. Open your legs to an open V shape (à la seconde), keeping your legs straight, as far as you can manage without feeling pain. Remember, please, do not force.

f. Stretch your body to one side, bending over that leg, then return to the center and stretch in the same way to the other side, over the other leg, flexing and pointing the feet once stretched to each side.

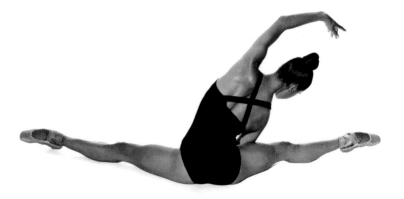

g. Sit up again and stretch forward. Now sit up and draw your legs toward each other along the floor, so that you finish with both legs straight out in front of you.

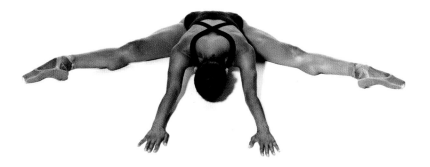

h. Finish with erect posture and a positive attitude.

16. Balancing Adagio

"Adagio" refers to slow movement in the ballet technique. As much as the adagio is about flexibility, strength, and fluidity in the movement, learning this exercise on the floor will give you an advantage before approaching it standing. On the floor you acquire a sense of balance and where your weight should be in order to leverage it to make your legs appear higher and more extended in opposition to your upper body.

This exercise should be done slowly to improve balance, alignment, abdominal strength, and stamina.

a. Start by sitting with your legs together on the floor in front of you.

b. Lift your legs into the air by bending your knees, holding the backs of your thighs with your hands with your legs still bent and parallel to each other.

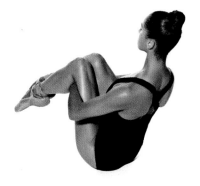

c. Leaning back, with your back straight and the backs of your thighs (hamstrings) leaning into your hands, slowly lengthen both legs into the air until they are fully straight, making you into a V shape.

d. Bend your knees so the tips of your toes touch the floor. Now do the same with each leg, alone, keeping the tips of the toes of your other leg poised on the floor.

e. Repeat the sequence, beginning with the other leg, when doing the single-leg section.

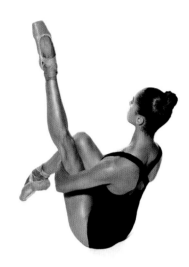

17. Grand Battement

"Grand battement" means "large kick." When doing a standing ballet barre, this is usually the last exercise you do while holding on to the barre before you move into the center of the room to dance without the barre's support. By the time you've gone through the sequence of technical exercises to get to the grands battements, you are extremely warm and have the flexibility to kick your legs high and long, preparing you for big jumps such as grands jetés.

This movement is good for elongating the muscles and freeing the hip joints, while maintaining stable postural alignment.

Do not be surprised if your legs do not go high to the back at first. Once you have learned to get the energy flowing through your whole body and out your legs without breaking at the waist, your legs will go higher.

a. Begin lying on your back in first position with your toes pointed (heels together, toes outward). With your arms at your sides and your palms facing down, use honest turnout (this is a rotation from the tops of the legs, without force, keeping the alignment of the core stable), en dehors, taut, as if jumping with the whole body in the air.

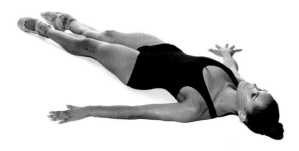

b. Kick four times in each direction—four grands battements front with the right leg, four front with the left leg—returning back to first position before each grand battement.

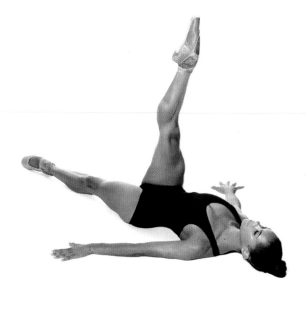

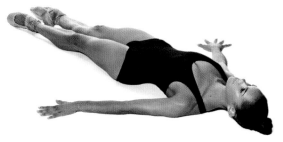

c. Then do four grands battements to the side with your right leg, and four to the side with your left leg. Move nothing but your working leg, keeping the back of your standing leg (the leg straight down on the floor) pressing into the floor.

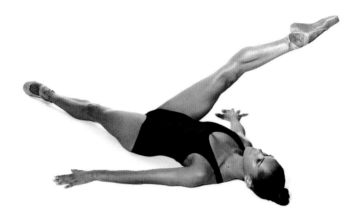

d. The back of your body should use the floor as a partner, but without force, as is the attitude throughout.

e. Because your legs are both elongated in this exercise, your lower back does not touch the floor in first position, although only the back of your waist, not your ribs, is off the floor.

f. Repeat the grands battements on your stomach, with your palms placed on top of each other and your forehead lying on the back of your top hand.

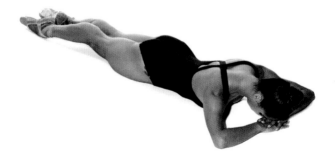

g. Perform four grands battements to the back with your right leg, four back with your left leg; four to the side with your right leg, four to the side with your left leg. Return back to first position before each grand battement.

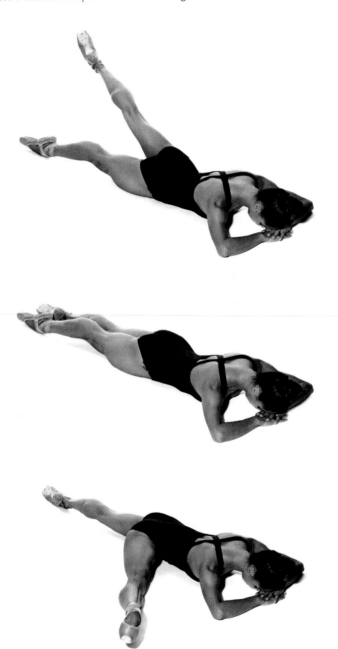

h. When kicking to the side, do not let go of the stability through the standing side, which should not move, allowing the alignment of the leg and the hip to be unbroken. Remain stable while one leg kicks.

i. Don't forget to use equal energy through both the standing and working legs, shooting out through the toes, at all times.

18. Finale

This is the final exercise of floor barre, as opposed to standing ballet barre, where grands battements come last. Finale is an incredible end to floor barre. I remember approaching finale for the first time and feeling so warm, and my body so placed, that I felt I could jump right off the floor. This exercise is another preparation for jumps (petit allegro, or small jumps), as is grands battements.

When doing this exercise, your position on the floor should emit an energy through the body, just as if you were standing or jumping in the air.

a. Begin in first position with flexed feet while lying on your back. Place your arms on the floor, to the sides, below the shoulders at a level that feels comfortable to you.

b. Slide your stretched legs along the floor, moving sideways in opposite directions, four times away from each other, stopping briefly between slides, and then four times toward each other, back to first position.

c. Next open your legs slightly away from each other with one motion rather than four small ones, and then pull them toward each other in one motion, returning to first position, as if the backs of your legs were magnetized. Do this sequence four times.

d. Repeat this series of steps two or four times.

e. Do the same exercise lying on your stomach, with your hands under your forehead, with the back of your neck elongated, and with energy shooting through the top of your head.

f. Make isometric use of the floor, not changing the length of all links and the center of the body while moving, whether on the back or the stomach, so as to gain length and strength faster and cleaner than a standing method. Pressing your body to the floor, using it in an isometric way, will help alignment with strength, length, and assurance, whether on the back or on the stomach.

g. Remember, your position on the floor should send an energy through your body just as if you were standing or jumping.

19. Stretch

In ballet, we wait to stretch when the body is thoroughly warm after an entire session at the barre. Stretching at this point is beneficial for both elongation and cooling down.

Every body is unique, requiring its own stretch, its own releases, and its own cooldowns. The same body may also require different stretches on different days. If you are very supple and loose, and you know how to do the splits correctly, this would be a good time to do them:

a. While sitting, bend forward over both legs lengthened in front of you, then opened (without force) to either side of the body. This is with the legs in second position.

b. Reach forward and stretch toward the floor, then bend over the right leg and then the left leg. Keep the backs of both legs and buttock cheeks pressed equally to the floor and bend at the waist without bending the knees to stretch the calves and the hamstrings.

c. Now lie on your stomach, legs lengthened, parallel to each other, separated and turned out.

d. Slowly push up into a back bend (back stretch), beginning with your head, bending one vertebra at a time.

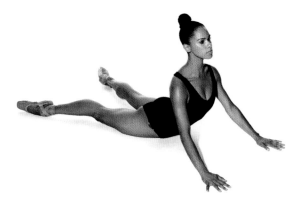

e. When coming down from the back bend, reach forward with the front of your chest (sternum) slowly until you reach the floor again, one vertebra at a time, head descending last. If you have no injuries or issues with your knees, push back and sit on your heels, with your heels remaining together under your buttocks, and put your head on the floor for relaxation. This helps to stretch the back in the opposite direction from the back bend, relieving any tension.

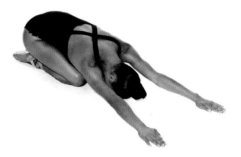

20. Stand

This exercise took me a couple of years to do after having my tibia surgery. It feels so awesome to be able to accomplish this now!

a. If at all possible, without putting your hands on the floor, find your way from the floor to a standing position.

b. While sitting, with both legs together and bent in a steady position, propel your upper body forward over your knees, pushing into your feet and straightening your knees to stand.

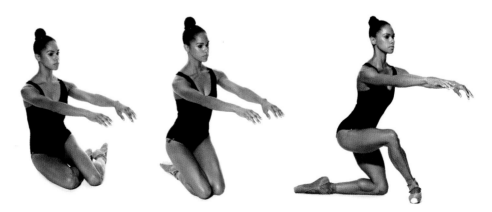

c. If you cannot manage this at first, keep looking for a way. You can try starting in the sitting position with one leg crossed in front of the other. Push your upper body forward to gain a little momentum and stand up, pushing onto the leg crossed in front.

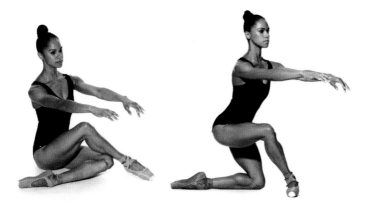

d. There is more than one way to do this correctly and gracefully. From this point forward, never get up from the floor by pushing off with your arms or allowing your shoulders to rise while doing so, even at home, when no one is watching! Once new muscle memory is created, this will become easy and natural.

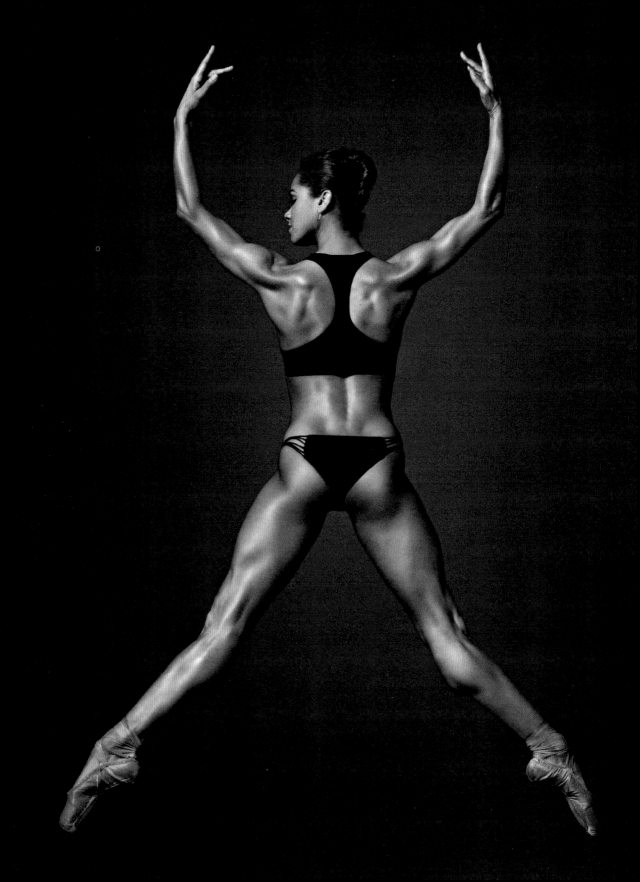

Chapter 6

TAKE CENTER STAGE

started taking floor barre class after developing six stress fractures to my tibia. I began to train in this technique a couple of months before my surgery, and once I had recovered completely and could stand again at the ballet barre, having my muscles trained and prepared by doing floor barre made me feel as though I had never stopped dancing.

Starting on the floor really prepares you to stand with a better trained body. But whether lying on the floor or standing on your feet, dancing shares the same general rules. Here are some important points about form:

a. Legs bend at three joints—the ankles, knees, and hips. When doing pliés (leg bends) keep the knees over the second and third toes. Never allow the knees to bend in front of the big toes. And do not tuck under! (Again, tucking under is gripping the buttock muscles, directing the tip of the tailbone forward.) Instead we want an uplifted feeling in the hip bones, while the tailbone points down toward the floor, not between the legs.

b. Next, shoulders should line up with the hip bones, the knees, and the cou-de-pied (the front of the ankle as it meets with the top of the foot) stacked one over the other: shoulders, hips, knees, cou-de-pied.

c. Your eyes generally should peer out right at eye level, or slightly above eye level.

d. Keep your weight over the balls of your feet, rather than sitting into your heels. This will allow you to move without first shifting your weight forward to travel, to rise onto your toes (relevé), or to jump.

Do the floor barre movements (Chapter 5) first, as a warm-up for these standing exercises. The more often you do these, the more proficient you will become. I suggest a minimum of twice a week, and six times a week wouldn't be too much. Whatever rhythm you start with, even if you don't have the time or energy to initially do the entire range of exercises, do what you can and build from there. The more you do, the more you will want to do.

Feel free to try these exercises holding on to a barre or the back of a chair—something stable—if you don't feel ready to do them freestanding.

Now that you know the proper form and pace, let's get moving!

1. BALLET WALK

Walking and running are two of the hardest things to learn in ballet and to make appear natural. As simple as the walks seem, you are training all of the small muscles in your feet and around your ankles to support your entire body and make as little noise as possible while you appear to be seamlessly floating. Here, we make use of the postural alignment and the flex and point of the floor barre, as we step toe, ball, heel.

    a. Walk by stepping and articulating through your toes, the ball of your foot, and then your heel, one foot after the other in the same manner. Begin slowly so you can master the toe, ball, heel walk. When it becomes easier, try going a bit faster, as long as it seems natural. You can practice walking around at home in this manner. The more you walk this way, the more natural it will become. Walking to music will give you a good tempo.

    b. Keep your back and posture erect, lengthening through the back of your neck. Keep your arms in second position, raised at your sides, slightly rounded. Your elbows should always remain slightly below your shoulders. Make sure your wrists are lower than your elbows. Remember, you want to make this way of walking look as comfortable and fluid as possible.

2. DEMI-PLIÉ

"Demi-plié" means "half bend," but to a dancer, it means to bend as far as you can go without releasing the heels from the floor. It's typically the first thing you do in ballet class at the barre. It's done in each of the five positions of the feet. The demi-plié prepares you for a full plié, also called a grand plié. In more advanced ballet classes, one may change the order of first and second position because second position is a wider, more open stance and it's easier to start with opening the hips in second position plié.

a. Let's start our demi-pliés in first position. Prepare for your first position by starting with your feet together, parallel to each other. Slide your toes and the front of your feet along the ground and allow your toes to open as far as they naturally go without forcing them.

b. Don't allow your knees to be affected. Remember your form. Your knees should be lined up over your toes. This will keep your joints safe.

c. If you do this exercise lying down, your knees should be pointed in the same direction as your toes. This rule applies to all of the positions. Turnout should come from the opening of your hips, not from forcing your toes out. Your bottom should remain in line with and right under your hips, not behind your hips or tucked under, pushing your pubic bone forward and causing your pelvis to tuck.

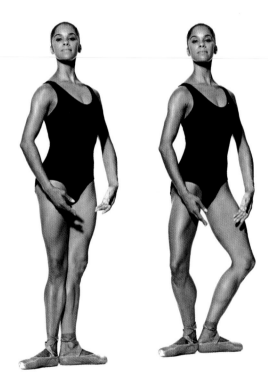

d. In first position, heels together and toes pointed out, bend your knees only as far as you can while keeping your heels on the floor. Once your heels come off the floor, that is considered to be a grand plié.

e. Do four demi-pliés in each position with your arms in fifth position en bas (down).

f. Do four demi-pliés in second position (feet pointed in the same direction as in first position with about one of your own feet's distance between the heels) with your arms in second position. Your arms are out to the sides, angled down and forward, with your palms facing forward. The rule for holding your arms is: shoulders, elbows, wrists, and fingers, in descending order.

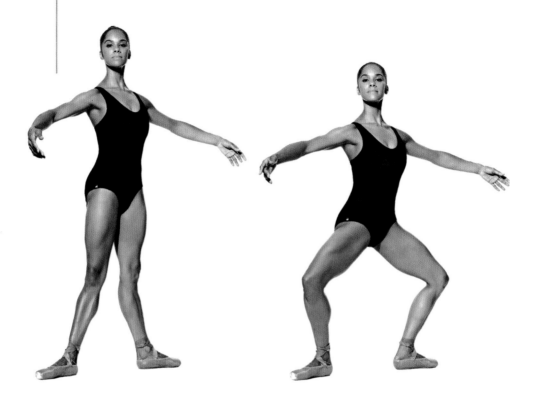

g. Do four demi-pliés in third position (one foot placed in front of the other so that the heel of the front foot is near the arch of the other). The toes of both feet should point away from each other, toward the side walls.

h. Then do four demi-pliés in fourth position, with the arms again held in first position, fingers in front of the stomach. One foot is placed approximately six inches in front of the other, or the length of one of your own feet. The heel of the front foot is aligned with the toe of the back foot. (This last move is advanced and not safe for beginners to try to accomplish.)

i. Next, do four demi-pliés in fifth position, with arms in low fifth position, forming an oval with hands held a few inches in front of the legs. In fifth position your feet should form two parallel lines. The heel of the front foot should be in contact with the big toe of the other, and the heel of the back foot should be in contact with the last toe of the front foot. (This heel-to-toe position is for advanced students. Beginners and amateurs can hurt themselves trying to accomplish this. They should not force the turnout this way.)

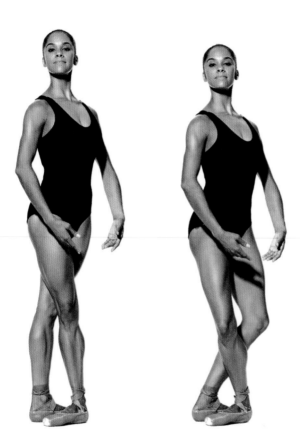

3. GRAND PLIÉ IN SECOND POSITION

"Grand plié" means "full plié," or a full bending of the knees. Throughout the movement, the pelvis should be kept neutral, the back straight and aligned with the heels, the legs turned out, and the knees over the feet. The transition from standing to knees fully bent should be fluid. Doing grand plié in second position, the heels never lift from the floor, unlike grands pliés in the other positions.

A purpose of the grand plié is to warm up the ankles and stretch the calves.

a. Place your feet apart, at least the length of one of your own feet between the heels.

b. Maintain an uplifted feeling as you bend your legs at the ankles, knees, and hips, keeping your knees pointing directly over your second and third toes. Again, never tuck your pelvis under. Keep your shoulders over your hips, over your knees, over your cous-de-pied (the neck of the foot, or the front of the ankles, where they meet the top of the feet). The arms too should be held in second position, which is held out to the sides, slightly in front of and below shoulder level, palms forward (facing the audience).

c. As soon as you've gone as far as possible, but not farther than the backs of thighs parallel to the floor, come up as smoothly as you went down.

d. Repeat and follow with a side bend left and side bend right. As a beginner, when you do the side bends, hold your arms out, in a circle, in front of your stomach, where the front ribs begin to open to the flesh of the stomach, as though you were hugging a tree. (This position of the arms is called an avant.) As you bend to the side and come back to center, keep your fingers directly in front of your stomach (with arms in second position, or à la seconde, but beginners may put their hands just below the hip bones to steady unstable hips and core). Keep everything still, from the waist down to the floor. Bend only the upper body to the side, keeping the shoulders in line with the hip bones.

e. If you have previous ballet training, you can follow the grands pliés à la seconde with port de bras à la seconde (meaning to the side).

4. BATTEMENT TENDU

"Tendu" means "stretched." For a battement tendu, you gradually extend the working leg to the front (tendu devant), side, or back, passing from flat foot to demi-pointe to pointe, where only the toes are touching the floor (tendu à terre). As you perform this exercise, feel the floor with your feet as you felt the floor with the part of your body that touched it while you were lying on it during the floor barre exercises. Using the floor this way sends messages of coordination throughout the body.

a. Stand erect, in a comfortable first position. Arms are in second position, as they were for Grands Pliés in second. With your knees stretched, without tension, brush the floor with the sole of your foot as you bring the demi-pointe (soles of the toes), then the tips of the toes to the floor in front, with your heel forward, but not forced.

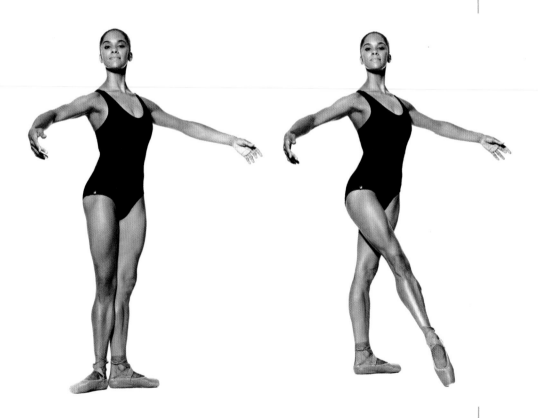

b. Then close first position by brushing the floor on the way in, passing through the demi-pointe and returning to first position.

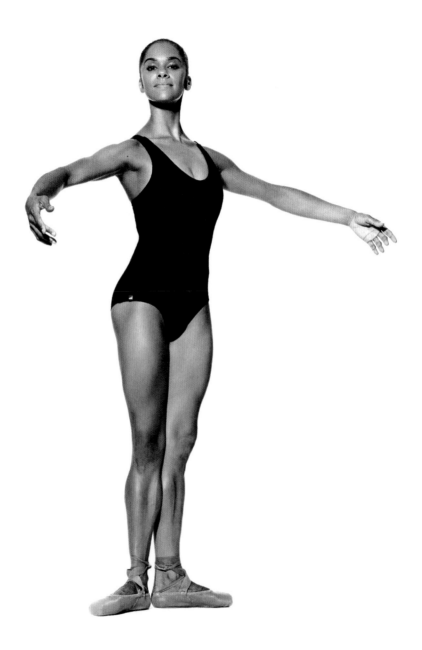

c. Do this two to four times each to the front, to the side, to the back, and to the side again (en croix, meaning front, side, back, side, in the shape of a cross).

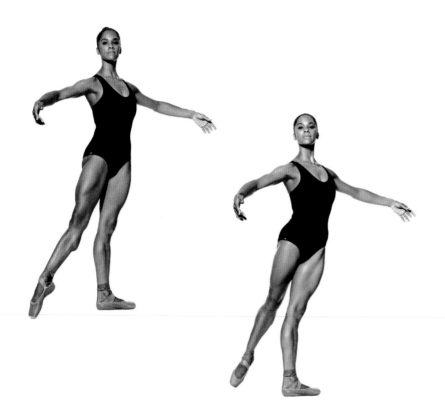

d. After you have done the tendus en croix, finish with a demi-plié in first position.

5. BATTEMENT DÉGAGÉ

"Dégagé" means "disengaged." The foot of the working leg sharply brushes over the floor through tendu, pointed two inches off the floor.

a. Begin in first position, arms held in second position. Brush through tendu (toe on the floor) and lift the pointed foot two inches off the floor, then return through tendu to first position.

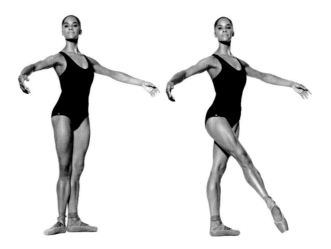

b. Do eight battements dégagés to each side. Feel the floor with your feet, sending the energy through the body, much like you did with your body lying on the floor during floor barre exercises.

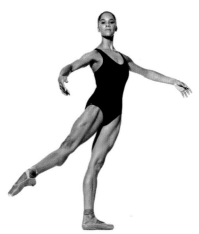

6. BATTEMENT EN CLOCHE

"En cloche" means "like a bell" and refers to brushing through first position from fourth devant (front) to fourth derrière (back), or from fourth derrière to fourth devant, with the upper body held upright. (The leg acts like the clapper of a bell as it rings.)

a. Begin in first position. Brush through first to dégagé front, then brush through first to dégagé back. Repeat four sets of front and back.

b. Finish with a demi-plié in first position.

7. ADAGIO

"Adagio" means "slowly," or at ease, walking forward two steps, toe, ball, heel.

a. Step into tendu back. Step into arabesque (standing on one leg with the other leg lifted behind, outstretched and pointed) with the arms en avant, in first position of the arms, just below shoulder level.

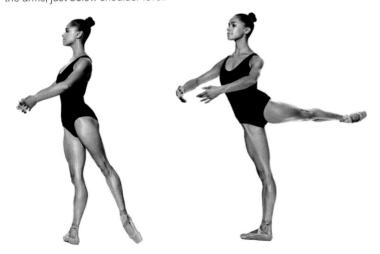

b. Bring the lifted leg forward and walk. Step into arabesque on the other leg.

c. Repeat four times, twice on each leg.

8. RELEVÉ

"Relevé" means "raised," or lifted, and describes the position when you rise onto the balls of your feet (demi-pointe) or onto the toes (pointe) of one or both feet.

    a. Begin in first position. Demi-plié, then stretch your knees and rise onto demi-pointe (relevé). Repeat this three times and hold on the count of four. When done to music, the counts are to the timing of the music.

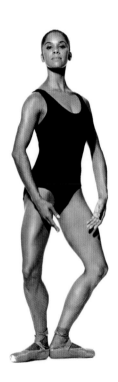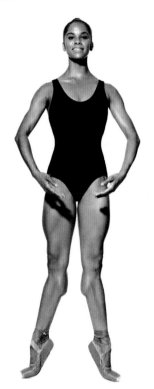

    b. Repeat once. When you get stronger, you may do four repetitions.

Remember to hold your posture as you did when you were lying on the floor for floor barre exercises. The flexing and pointing also prepare and strengthen your ankles to allow you to stand on demi-pointe (or en pointe, if you are an advanced dancer).

9. JUMP

If your body is healthy and strong enough to jump, begin in first position. A good demi-plié prepares and finishes every jump. In the air, your legs will be stretched, with pointed feet.

a. Do eight small jumps in first position, jumping only high enough to point the feet in the air. Then land, toe, ball, heel, to a demi-plié after every jump. Your arms should remain in second position.

b. Échappé (meaning "escaped") is a movement done from a closed first position to an open second position. In an échappé sauté (jump), a dancer takes a deep plié followed by a jump in which the legs "escape" into second position, landing in demi-plié.

c. Jump from first to second position and back to first: Begin in first position, demi-plié. Jump and land, toe, ball, heel, in second position, demi-plié.

d. Jump again, bringing your legs together in the air, then landing in first position, toe, ball, heel, to demi-plié.

e. Jumps may be repeated more slowly and higher. The arms should remain in the en bas position. Whenever the arms are rounded to form an oval, they are in fifth position. There is a fifth position en bas (arms down, framing your torso), or fifth en avant (arms above your head, framing your face).

10. SPOTTING EXERCISE

a. Stand in an easy first position.

b. Put your hands on your hip bones with the elbows pointing to the sides.

c. Choose a point to spot in front of you, at eye level or slightly higher.

d. Begin by turning slowly, with tiny steps in one direction, keeping your eyes focused on the spot you've chosen.

e. When you are about to lose sight of your spot, snap your head around to the other side to see it again as quickly as possible.

f. Continue turning in the same direction, the same way, slowly increasing the speed.

g. Do not lose sight of your spot, or you will get dizzy. This is the secret dancers use to keep from getting dizzy when they turn.

h. Repeat the spotting exercise to the other side.

11. PORT DE BRAS

"Port de bras" means "carriage of the arms," and this exercise is for the movement of the arms (and in some schools the upper body) to different positions.

The phrase "port de bras" is used in some schools and parts of the world to indicate a bending forward, backward, or circling of the body at the waist, generally to be followed by bringing the upper body back to center or upright again (port de bras forward, port de bras back, circular port de bras, grand port de bras). Bending at the waist is otherwise known as camber.

We do port de bras on the floor by using the hands and arms on the floor to connect and coordinate the whole body. Lying on your back, lift the arms above the shoulders, palms down on the floor, pushing the core off the floor with a straight back, coming to a seated position, then bending over the legs, then returning to a seated position. Use that same feeling while doing this exercise standing.

a. Begin standing with your legs parallel. Send energy down through your legs, into the floor. Roll your head forward, down through your spine, one vertebra at a time, as far as you can go without bending your knees.

b. Then bend your legs in demi-plié and stretch them, lengthening the backs of your legs.

c. Now roll up with the same slow tempo you used to roll down.

d. Port de bras can be repeated in an easy first position this time, keeping the posture erect and bending at the hips, curling forward only when you can go no farther with a straight back.

e. Come up again with a stretched back on elongated legs, which should continue to push away the floor, returning to a standing position with good posture.

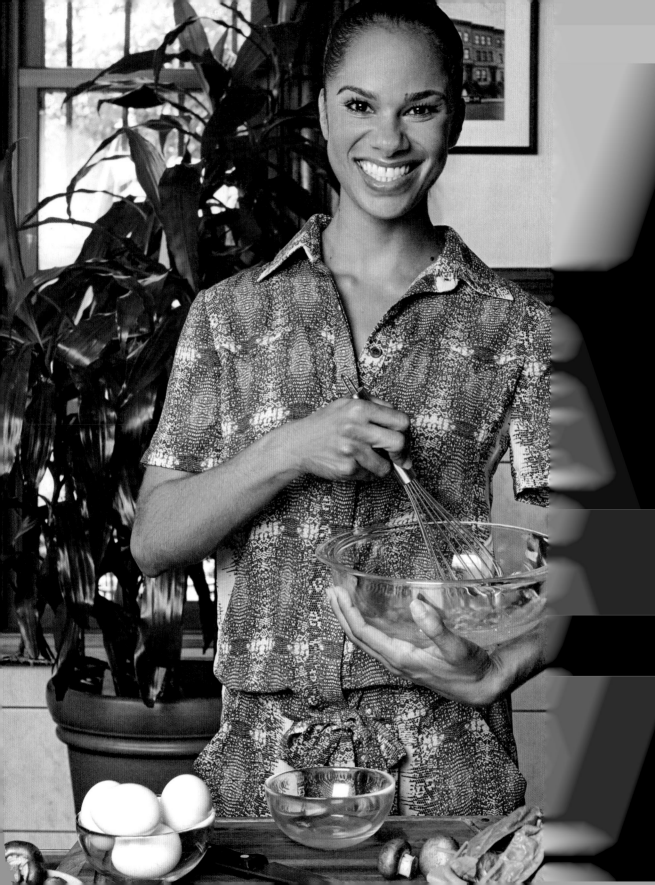

PART 3

Meals

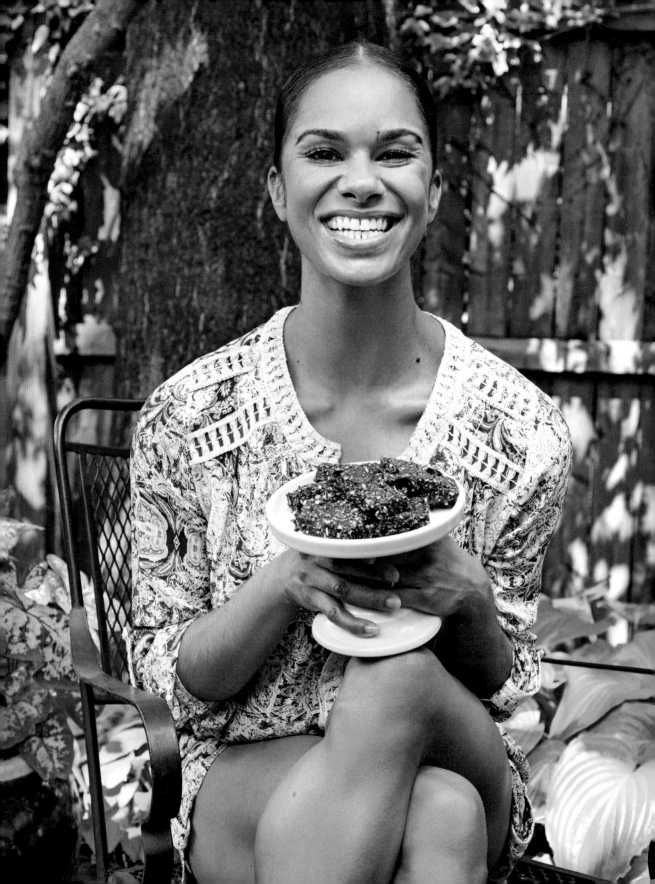

Chapter 7

THE MAGIC OF FAT

One of the greatest secrets I have learned over the course of my career is that fat—eating it, absorbing it, and burning it for energy—is key to building the muscle and providing the strength so important for ballerinas and all elite athletes to perform at such a high level for hours, day in and day out.

Fat will work the same way for you. Eating healthy fats, along with my fitness program, can create body-curving muscle, which is vital to an efficient metabolism and calorie burn. Fat will also provide the energy you need to continue sculpting your ballerina body and to engage in all the other activities and passions that matter to you and make your life worthwhile.

I know that it may sound confusing that you should eat fat to stay lean. When my body began to fill out in my late teens, I thought that I would have to radically pare my diet, giving up my favorite foods for a bland diet of rice cakes and skim milk. It seemed like an impossible regimen to stick with. I soon found out that the truth was that I would have to make some sacrifices, but fat—the good kind, found in fish and nuts, avocados and seeds—wouldn't have to be one of them.

THE TRUTH ABOUT FAT

I used to bury my hurt in a box of Krispy Kremes.

When I entered the world of ballet, I was told by some that I was too old to be a beginner. Others thought my skin color was an obstacle. But my body—my knees, which jutted backward, large feet, narrow torso, and tiny head—was deemed to be perfect. It was the combination of angles and proportions that the choreographer George Balanchine said added up to the ideal ballerina.

Then, seemingly overnight, parts of my body changed. My waifish figure had acquired womanly curves. I gained ten pounds over several months, and while I didn't continue to put on weight, I wasn't losing any either. And my instructors had told me, in the code-speak of dance, that I needed to "lengthen," or slim down.

There was a Krispy Kreme bakery near my apartment in Manhattan, and so late at night, anxious about the need to fine-tune my body and in the dark about what to do and where to turn, I would call and place an order. They weren't willing to drop off a mere one or two doughnuts. In fact, the bakery delivered only to businesses. So, I would get a whole box of sugar-crusted pastries dropped at my door. And I'd sit on my couch and eat the whole thing.

The next morning, I'd feel heavy—in my body and in my spirit, because I knew that those late-night binges were setting me back. I didn't have the energy I needed to rehearse eight hours a day, and my body wasn't as in tune as it needed to be to perform as an elite athlete.

I knew I had to make a change. And eventually I found great support on this new journey, from one person in particular: Olu, the man I had begun dating and who eventually became my husband. Having someone I trusted there to encourage and motivate me was invaluable, and it helped launch me onto a new path.

Olu was a pescatarian. He was raised eating fish as his main protein source. After hearing about the benefits of a fish-centered diet, and being the type of person I am, I dove in headfirst, becoming a pescatarian overnight. I wouldn't necessarily recommend going cold turkey like I did. I had dreams of bacon and giant hamburgers for months! But I felt amazing. My energy level skyrocketed, and the formula for long, lean muscles that I'd been searching for finally came together. I know that cutting out red meat, chicken, and pork is not for everyone, and it may be best to wean yourself off those foods gradually. But for me, it seemed to be the final missing link.

I've since come to understand that fat burns fat. To put it simply, you need certain fats to cancel out the stubborn bulges that pop up around your belly, your thighs, and your hips. But it's not the kind of fat loaded into the doughnuts and corn chips I used to love so much. It's the good fat—full of omega-3s—that flows through fish like tuna, sardines, and my favorite, salmon.

The more I ate of the good stuff, and the more I left the doughnuts alone, the more I noticed my arms and legs getting leaner and my stomach becoming more taut. My workouts also started to feel more explosive, turbocharged by my growing stamina. I'd discovered the science behind the changes I'd experienced firsthand in my own body.

Without new fat—either gleaned from foods that we eat or created in the liver—old fat already present around the posterior or tummy makes a beeline for the liver, where it lurks and builds up. But when new fat appears, it turns on an important protein that ramps up the metabolism—boosting energy and incinerating calories.

I also began to try to figure out what exercises worked best at getting my body to function at its peak. I began to notice that when I used weights, I built up muscle very quickly, bulking up my frame and moving my figure further away from a lean silhouette. So I cut those exercises out of my regimen. Again, it turned out that what I had discovered by trial and error was also backed by science. I didn't need extra weights to boost my muscles. The fat that I was getting from my evolving diet was sharpening my muscle tone with my normal dance workouts and was also helping my muscles to heal and grow.

So that means the muscle you build with the Ballerina Body plan will have multiple benefits. Not only are you reshaping your physique, but when you have more muscle, your body burns fat and calories more efficiently, especially when you work out. And a succulent piece of fish, drizzled with lemon juice, or chopped in a salad, will help to sculpt your muscles even more and ignite those calories even when you're resting. It's a win, win, win.

Fat Makes You Happy *and* Fills You Up

Certain types of fish, and other omega-3-packed items like flaxseed oil, are kinds of wonder foods, experts say. Not only do they burn fat and build muscle, but omega-3s also can pump up your levels of serotonin, that natural, feel-good brain chemical that also gets a boost when you meditate or exercise. And when your mood gets a lift, so do your motivation and willpower, helping you to push that gallon of ice cream to the back of the freezer, or, even better, to bypass it altogether when you're making your way down the grocery store aisle.

Fat also fills you up. I've realized that firsthand.

When I get home from a long day of classes and rehearsals, I can't wait to curl up on the couch and have a snack. Or, depending on how much or little I ate earlier, I may be in the mood for a full meal.

When I was a teenager, before I joined ABT, my favorite dinner was shrimp scampi, with the shrimp swimming in a bowl of fragrant, garlicky, buttery noodles. Later, after I moved to New York, I also loved the succulent, falling-off-the-bone ribs at Dallas BBQ. And my best friend and I were willing to take a forty-five-minute subway ride to get those cheddar biscuits at Red Lobster. We were ecstatic when the chain finally opened a spot closer to where we lived in Manhattan!

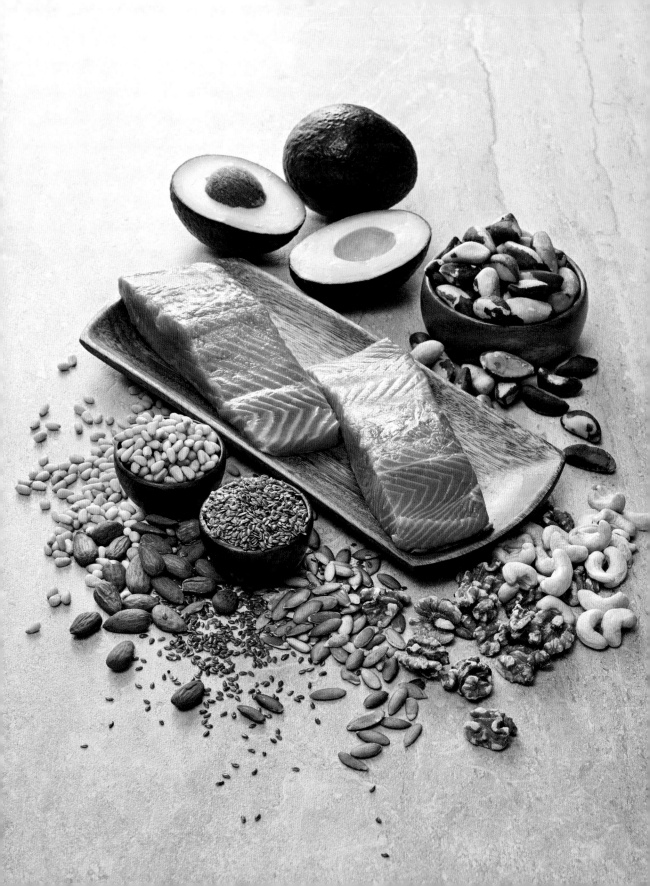

But the next morning, the elation I felt while we were having dinner had long faded as I stood in class feeling lethargic and staring at a reflection that was heavier than it needed to be to do what my body needed to do.

Nutrition wasn't part of ABT's repertoire, and I couldn't afford to hire a dietitian. I was fumbling in my search to pinpoint what meal plan was best for my health and endurance, but I knew that devouring a heaping plate of pasta or a sugar-crusted dessert late at night couldn't be a part of it.

I kept building out my new menu. Along with a small portion of fish, I began to fill my plate with vegetables when I wanted something more substantial, or I'd grab a handful of pistachios when I felt a small snack was enough. I soon noticed that even though I was eating much less, I'd feel full and go to bed satisfied. I was also no longer feeling bloated or tired when I got up the next morning. And faster than I'd expected, I was able to wean myself off of the snack foods I'd craved so much. I rarely wanted them anymore.

It turns out that all those good fats found in some nuts and fish fill you up and act like a natural appetite suppressant, quelling the urge to overindulge in foods that you should eat sparingly, if at all. Fat, you see, doesn't digest very quickly. It lingers in your digestive tract longer than most nutrients. That leaves you feeling satiated, not just right after your breakfast, lunch, or dinner, but for up to two hours later. And that, in turn, can lead to weight loss.

Fat Is Energizing and Helps You Absorb More Nutrition

With all we have going on, heading to classes, commuting to work, parenting children, hanging out with friends, we need as much energy as we can get. When I'm not rehearsing at ABT, I've got errands to run and people to see, and I realize that it's food that provides the fuel to carry me through, so it's good to know what will give me the biggest boost. It's not just nutrient-packed carbohydrates like blueberries, oatmeal, and tomatoes that flood your body with energy. Fat is a powerful kick-starter as well. In fact, a gram of fat has double the energy of a gram of carbs.

And certain nutrients, namely, vitamins A, D, E, and K, can't be absorbed by your body without fat, and that can lead to dry skin, weak bones, achy muscles, and fatigue. But when you're absorbing these vitamins as you're eating some good fats in your diet, they can help to keep your weight under control.

Fat Fights Inflammation

As a dancer, I face the risk of injury every day. As is true for other athletes, there's the ever-present possibility of sprained ankles, pulled hamstrings, and fractured bones. But fat works as an anti-inflammatory nutrient, enabling your body to be more resistant to injury so you can keep up your workout without being sidelined. And when chronic inflammation—a process that can also interfere with your body's ability to burn fat—does occur, a fat-based diet helps to manage and resolve it. So fat is a source of prevention *and*, potentially, a part of the cure.

FAT MYTHS

Still, it can be hard to overcome old perceptions. Fat is shrouded in so many misperceptions that most people may not realize that it's actually a vital nutrient. We've talked about many of the ways that it helps and heals our bodies, but to banish any remaining mental hurdles to eating it, let's shatter some of the myths about fat once and for all.

Myth 1: If You Eat Fat, You'll Get Fat

The reality is that rather than becoming heavier from eating fat, depending on which fats you focus on, the opposite can occur.

When I was contemplating what menu would give me the most energy and help me to have a leaner frame, foods marked low-fat piqued my interest. At the grocery store, or even when I was out at a restaurant, there seemed to be a low-fat option for virtually every snack, drink, or entrée, from low-cal yogurt to lower-carb versions of bread.

If I grabbed a couple of low-fat yogurts, I felt that I was in the clear, feeding my sweet tooth, getting some bone-strengthening calcium, but keeping the calories to a healthy minimum because, after all, it was supposed to be low-fat. But I was falling into the same trap that snares so many of us. Because I figured fat was one of the main culprits when it came to putting on excess pounds, I believed that eating more of a supposedly healthier option wouldn't be a problem.

But often, those labels lull us into a false sense of comfort, and we wind up consuming more than we should. Then we are left feeling dissatisfied with the fit of our clothes, how

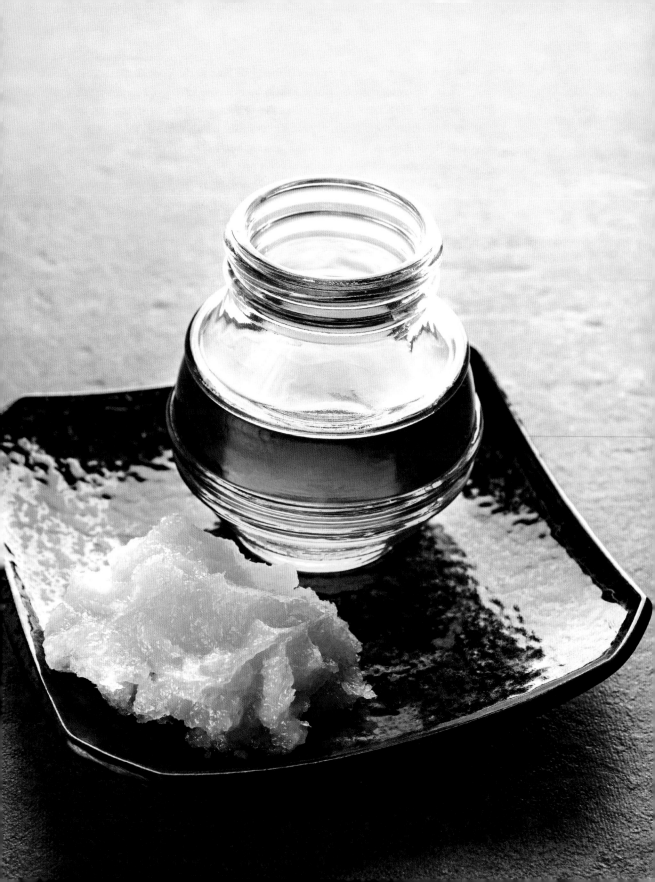

we look in the mirror, and the lack of energy we have to carry out all the tasks we need to handle. *Or* we eat more because it actually takes several servings for us to feel full.

A diet that is heavier in carbs, like rice or potatoes, is less satisfying than a diet that leans more on nuts, seeds, vegetables, and fish, which is possibly one of the reasons that the U.S. population, overall, is getting heavier, though we're eating less fat than we did in the past.

And while grabbing products labeled low-fat may seem like a simple way to identify what's best to eat, some of those foods may actually be detrimental to our health. Low-fat cookies or cheeses, for instance, might be loaded with sugar or salt to enhance the taste. So eating more protein, paring back the carbs, and following the Ballerina Body menu, which emphasizes fish and olive oil, can be a better plan (you'll learn more about what to eat in Chapter 8).

Myth 2: Fat Is a Toxin That Leads to Heart Disease and Cancer

That's certainly what I, like many people, used to believe. But when it comes to toxic nutrients, sugar is actually the biggest problem. The heart relies on fat for fuel. And the bottom line is that not all foods containing saturated fats are created equally—some may be a safeguard against coronary heart disease, and when they are swapped out in favor of foods containing high-fructose corn syrup or some other sugars, the chance for developing heart disease may actually grow.

Myth 3: Fat Is a Poor Source of Energy

Fat is actually an energy-packed nutrient. With 9 calories per gram, it provides more than twice the energy—or calories—found in a gram of carbohydrate or even a gram of protein.

And when your muscles are crying out for energy, especially after you exercise, fat is the source that is most abundantly available—because when it's stored in your body, that's essentially what fat is.

Myth 4: All Fats Are Bad

By now, I hope it's clear that fats are actually, mostly, great. But there are a few types that you do need to steer clear of.

First there are hydrogenated fats, which are most often found in white bread, corn oil, and some sweets, like the doughnuts I used to love. They may extend a food's shelf life in the pantry, and they can prevent it from melting at room temperature, but it's bad for our health, especially when some of those fats turn into something known as trans-fatty acids, which can lead to heart disease, high cholesterol, and breast cancer.

Concerns about the toxicity of trans fats led the U.S. Food and Drug Administration to declare in June 2015 that partially hydrogenated oil is generally not considered safe, spurring the food industry to largely stop using it. But hydrogenated and trans fats are definitely still out there. You can take matters into your own hands by checking labels and avoiding fast food and the commercially baked cookies, biscuits, and cakes that may contain a lot of trans fats.

One more thing: Watch out for omega-6 fats—which are found in oils made from sources like sunflowers and corn. Eating *more* omega-6 fats than omega-3s may cause you to gain weight. So, as in all other aspects of our lives, balance is key.

A NEW WAY OF EATING

FOR A NEW WAY OF LIVING

Many of us can stick to a diet for a few days, a few weeks, maybe even a few months. But if an eating plan is too unrealistic, restrictive, or unappetizing, we'll abandon it eventually, and any positive results we get will be as fleeting as the time we spent depriving ourselves.

That's why the Ballerina Body plan is not a temporary fix, but a whole new way of eating that is diverse and delicious enough that you will be motivated to make it an integral part of your life. Of course, eating more vegetables than you're used to and cutting back on soda or sugar may take some adjustment. But I truly believe that your palate can learn to crave new textures and flavors. And I think that when you experience your energy level improving, see your muscles growing more defined, and feel your mood get a boost, you'll embrace this new diet wholeheartedly. It's a meal plan that tastes as good as it makes you feel, and that should be worth sticking with.

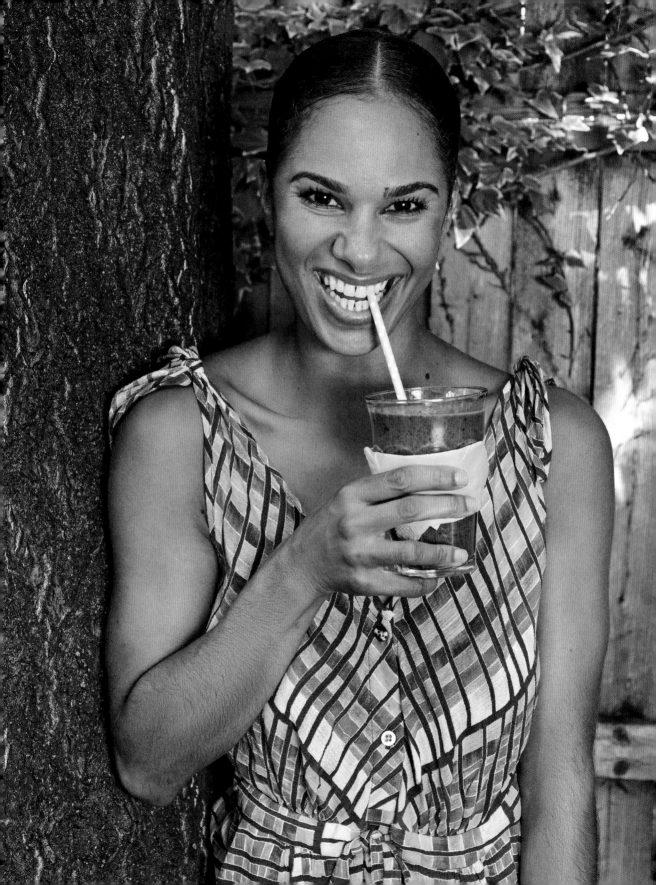

Chapter 8

EATING
FOR ENERGY

The Ballerina Body meals and recipes are higher in fat than those in some other eating plans because fat is an essential nutrient that provides us with numerous benefits. But the Ballerina Body meal plan includes and highlights other quality foods as well that our bodies will use to accelerate our energy, sculpt our muscles, burn off fat, and mold our physiques into the shape we desire.

There are two broad categories of food that you will get to eat. First are the **Act 1** foods, which are the main ingredients of all your meals and are the primary suppliers of the fats you need to keep your body in fat-burning mode. Act 1 foods include three food groups:

- Animal proteins.
- Plant fats.
- Beneficial oils.

The second broad category is **Act 2** foods. These foods play a vital supporting role in your diet:

- Fibrous vegetables, which are high in fiber and low in calories. Eat as many of these as you want.
- Fruits, including dried fruits.
- Fibrous starches, including beans, lentils, potatoes, sweet potatoes, yams, beets, turnips, parsnips, carrots, corn, grains such as rice,

oats, quinoa, and others; tofu; whole-grain bread, muffins, and bagels; and whole wheat pasta.

All these food groups and categories contribute different nutrients and assume different tasks that are crucial to stoking our energy and boosting the functions vital to improving and maintaining our health. Let's take a look at each category.

ACT 1 FOODS

Animal Proteins

Animal proteins have multiple benefits.

- They provide building blocks called amino acids for manufacturing muscle—that's key for chiseling your body shape and maintaining a revved-up metabolism.
- They contain fats that stimulate fat burning, particularly fish with their powerful omega-3s.
- They keep you feeling full longer thanks to their fat and protein content.
- They have important vitamins and minerals. From dairy to lean meats and fish, animal proteins are a wellspring of the vitamins and minerals we need, and at times they expedite how quickly we are able to absorb them. For example, the mineral zinc is integral to the functioning of the immune system and helps to break down carbohydrates. But it is harder for us to get the zinc we need from plants and vegetables than from protein. I prefer fish as my main protein source, and I don't eat meat, but if you do eat meat, pork and beef actually have even more zinc than fish does. Chicken is another key source. Dairy products, meanwhile, are bursting with bone-health boosters such as calcium, and milk, eggs, and fish have plenty of B vitamins, which keep us energized.

Here are examples of the kinds of animal proteins to keep stocked in your kitchen.

Fish and Shellfish

Bass	Halibut*	Redfish	Shark
Bluefish	Herring*	Red snapper	Shrimp
Catfish	Lobster	Salmon, canned	Tilapia
Clams	Mackerel*	and drained, or	Trout
Cod	Mahimahi	fresh*	Tuna (fresh or
Crabmeat	Mussels	Sardines, packed in	low-sodium,
Flounder	Orange roughy	water, mustard,	packed in water)*
Grouper	Oysters	or tomato sauce*	Whitefish
Haddock	Perch	Scallops	

Nutritional benefits: Big plus: omega-3s. Those fish marked with an asterisk are especially high in this type of fatty acid, which is known to help the body burn fat and supply numerous other benefits.

Prep tips: Because we want to eke the most benefit out of our meals, we want to avoid frying fish in less-than-healthy oils. Try grilling, baking, poaching, or broiling instead.

How to shop: Wild instead of farm-raised fish may be the optimum way to go. Take, for instance, salmon. Wild salmon tends to be lower in calories, organic pollutants that can lead to illness, and saturated fat.

Then there's the matter of mercury. It's been recommended that women who are pregnant, new mothers, and young children stick to fish with lower mercury content, such as salmon, tilapia, cod, and tuna. Some larger fish, which are more likely to have higher amounts of mercury, are best left alone. Those include shark, king mackerel, tilefish, and swordfish. And if you enjoy albacore tuna, try not to eat more than 6 ounces a week.

Serving size: 4 to 5 ounces, or the size of your hand or a deck of cards.

Poultry

Chicken, ground	Chicken thighs, skin	Turkey, ground
Chicken breast,	removed	Turkey breast, light
skin removed	Cornish game hens	and dark meat

Nutritional benefits: When it comes to poultry, the juicy, dark meat in particular pops with zinc, a major booster for the immune system. Chicken also contains vitamin

B$_6$, which assists in the breakdown of carbs and protein, and selenium, an antioxidant that helps combat cancer. And poultry is chock-full of niacin, or vitamin B$_3$, which keeps the cells in top shape and may decrease the chance of getting heart disease.

Prep tips: Don't nip the nutritional benefits of poultry by dousing it in batter and deep-frying it in oil. Broil, bake, grill, or roast instead. Be careful not to undercook! That puts you at risk for salmonella poisoning and other unpleasant bacterial ailments. You can use a meat thermometer to make sure your chicken or turkey is cooked through. Look for a reading of at least 165°F.

How to shop: There's a dizzying array of options when it comes to buying poultry. They include natural, which means they don't have additives, free-range chickens, which are allowed to roam outside, birds that don't contain any antibiotics, and organic—a USDA certification that the poultry had a vegetarian, pesticide-free diet, among other qualifications.

Serving size: 4 to 5 ounces, or the size of your hand or a deck of cards.

Meats

Beef	Buffalo	Lamb	Veal
Beef, ground	Buffalo, ground	Pork	

Nutritional benefits: Contrary to what some may believe, meats are excellent fat burners. Besides the fact that they contain fat-destroying saturated fat, they also have plenty of the amino acid leucine, which is also found in fish and dairy products and helps you whittle down while maintaining calorie-burning muscle.

Prep tips: Baking, broiling, grilling, and roasting are the best ways to get the most nutritional value.

How to shop: As there are for poultry, there are various labels for beef, pork, and other meat, including grass-fed—meaning that the animals eat only what is foraged and are antibiotic-free, raised without exposure to hormones, and organic.

Serving size: 4 to 5 ounces, or the size of your hand or a deck of cards.

Dairy

Cottage cheese	Eggs	Goat cheese	Ricotta cheese
Cream cheese	Feta cheese	Hard cheese	Yogurt, full-fat

Nutritional benefits: Dairy products give you a package of essential nutrients, especially calcium, which is a bone-building mineral that dancers need, because it's not just our muscles that are constantly in motion, but also our bones.

During the time that I was performing as the Firebird, the six stress fractures that I suffered in my tibia nearly ended my career. It took months of grueling rehabilitation for me to be able to get back to dancing, and months more once I was back onstage to regain my dexterity and strength.

I also have hyperextended knees, which have given me a desirable line for ballet, but also make me more prone to injury. I needed to learn to retrain my body so that my muscles were supporting my bones in a healthier way, but I had to change more than just my ballet technique. Diet was key, and dairy has played a significant role.

Some people are lactose-intolerant, meaning that they have trouble breaking down the sugar naturally found in dairy foods. But that doesn't mean you can't enjoy those products. You shouldn't have a problem if you choose yogurt or cheese, lactose-free milk, or even dairy-free milks, such as almond, coconut, or rice milk, which can supply you with a dose of calcium.

And if you don't particularly care for dairy foods, that's okay too. On the Ballerina Body eating plan you don't have to consume foods that you don't like. It's important that you have a menu you enjoy so that you stick with the healthy eating plan. It's all about flexibility. So you can scratch dairy off the list if you choose. There are enough other options to allow you to choose your favorites and still boost your health and achieve a ballerina body.

Prep tips: Cheese, eggs, yogurt, and milk are delicious on their own, as snacks, and also in recipes. I'll often grab a cup of yogurt or cottage cheese for a tasty treat in the middle of the day.

Serving size: 1 egg; 6 ounces (about ⅔ cup) yogurt, cottage cheese, or ricotta cheese; ⅓ cup feta or goat cheese; 2 ounces hard cheese (about the size of a domino); 2 tablespoons cream cheese.

Plant Fats

Nuts have become my go-to snack. I keep a baggie or small container of them in my purse and my locker at ABT's rehearsal studio because I've found that they satisfy my hunger and give me a quick spike of energy.

It turns out that certain plant foods—from nuts to seeds to nut butters and avocados—are full of beneficial, fat-burning fats. Fruits, veggies, and some nuts, like almonds and pistachios, are also full of fiber, which helps control weight because fiber tends to make you feel full, so you consume less. Nuts in particular can be filling without adding on excess pounds.

Then there are all those phytonutrients, the compounds in greens, tomatoes, sprouts, and other foods that promote a strong heart, safeguard your vision, preserve bone strength, and guard against cancer. And avocados and olives are motherlodes of healthful properties. Both contain monounsaturated fats, which can help prevent the deposit of fat around your middle. Both foods are heart-healthy too.

Nuts

Almonds	Nut butters, any	legumes, though	Peanut butter
Brazil nuts	type	they are often	Pecans
Cashews	Peanuts (Peanuts	thought of as	Pine nuts
Macadamia nuts	are actually	nuts)	Walnuts

Serving size: a small handful or ⅛ cup nuts; 1 tablespoon nut butters.

Seeds

Flaxseeds	Sesame seeds	Tahini (sesame
Pumpkin seeds	Sunflower seeds	seed butter)

Serving size: a handful of seeds; 1 tablespoon seed butter.

Others

Avocado	Olives

Serving size: ½ avocado; 6 olives.

Nutritional benefits: Nuts and seeds are tiny packages of fiber, protein, and omega-3 fatty acids that are great for your heart. Avocados, meanwhile, are chock-full of potassium, B vitamins, and monounsaturated fats that together help to ward off illness, boost eye health, and control cholesterol.

Prep tips: These foods make for wonderful snacks or tasty toppings. Sprinkle a few nuts on top of your cereal, add some sunflower seeds to a salad, toss your avocado with some lemon juice, or spread almond butter on a stalk of celery.

How to store: Nuts and seeds can be preserved for several months in the refrigerator or even in the freezer. Nuts not encased in a shell should be packed in dry, sealed containers.

When it comes to preserving nut butters, store them in covered jars, tucked in the refrigerator or on a cool dry shelf in the pantry or kitchen cabinet.

Beneficial Oils

There are three oils that I love and that I feel are great additions to our diet.
- Olive oil
- Coconut oil
- Flaxseed oil

Olive Oil

This is one of my favorite oils to cook with. It adds richness to your dish but is a healthier alternative than butter. In fact, olive oil offers so many benefits that it might be easier to sum up what olive oil *doesn't* do.

Nutritional benefits: Olive oil, long linked to longevity in Mediterranean cultures, where it's a key ingredient in the diet, contains the antioxidant compounds known as polyphenols, which account for its many health benefits. Some of these polyphenols are unique—they can't be found in any other fruit or vegetable. Protecting your heart, fighting inflammation, warding off germs, and normalizing blood pressure are just a few of the tasks that olive oil performs.

Prep tips: Olive oil is flavorful and versatile. Use it to sauté fish or meat, drizzle it on vegetables, make it a dip for bread, or use it as a salad dressing.

How to shop: Here's a brief glossary of the different types.
- Virgin: Oil that's produced without chemicals or extreme heat.
- Extra-virgin: The top of the line, and the type recommended as the most nutritious. Its processing leads to less acidity.
- Cold-pressed: This is an outdated term that refers to a decades-old production technique that is not really used any longer.

How to store: Keep it sealed in a space away from sunlight or heat. You can put it in the refrigerator, but it's not necessary.

Serving size: 1 to 2 tablespoons daily.

Coconut Oil

Nutritional benefits: This is another of my favorite oils to cook with because it's so tasty. The statements about coconut oil have been all over the map, and a key knock against it is that it's very high in saturated fat. However, according to the Mayo Clinic, coconut oil's particular kind of fat is the energy-pumping lauric acid. And when it comes to causing cholesterol to spike, some research indicates that lauric acid is a lesser culprit than some other fats.

There are different varieties, including:

- Virgin: Oils that are derived from fresh coconut.
- Refined: These are the most common oils eaten around the globe; they undergo processes such as filtering or steaming. While some of the nutritional value may be lost through some of those treatments, the vital fats remain.

Prep tips: Bake with coconut oil instead of butter, use it to sauté fish and vegetables, or sprinkle a few drops on top of fruit.

How to shop: What you buy should depend on how much you love coconut. Virgin often has a stronger flavor than refined.

How to store: You can keep it in the pantry or the refrigerator.

Serving size: A single tablespoon of coconut oil can pack 117 calories. So if you want to add it to your diet, use it with a light touch.

Flaxseed Oil

Nutritional benefits: This oil contains 50 to 60 percent omega-3 fatty acids, so if you don't like fish, here's your omega-3-rich alternative. Those fatty acids mean flaxseed oil promotes healthy brain function and helps to lower the risk of heart disease. And flaxseed oil also has anti-inflammatory properties, which is the number one reason I like it, to keep potential swelling in check.

Prep tips: Flaxseed oil is not great for cooking, but it works well in pesto, hummus, and salad dressings.

How to shop: When choosing a flaxseed oil, go for the unfiltered varieties, which offer more nutrients.

How to store: Since it has a short shelf life, stash it in the fridge.

Serving size: One tablespoon of flaxseed oil has 120 calories, so like coconut oil, you might want to use it sparingly.

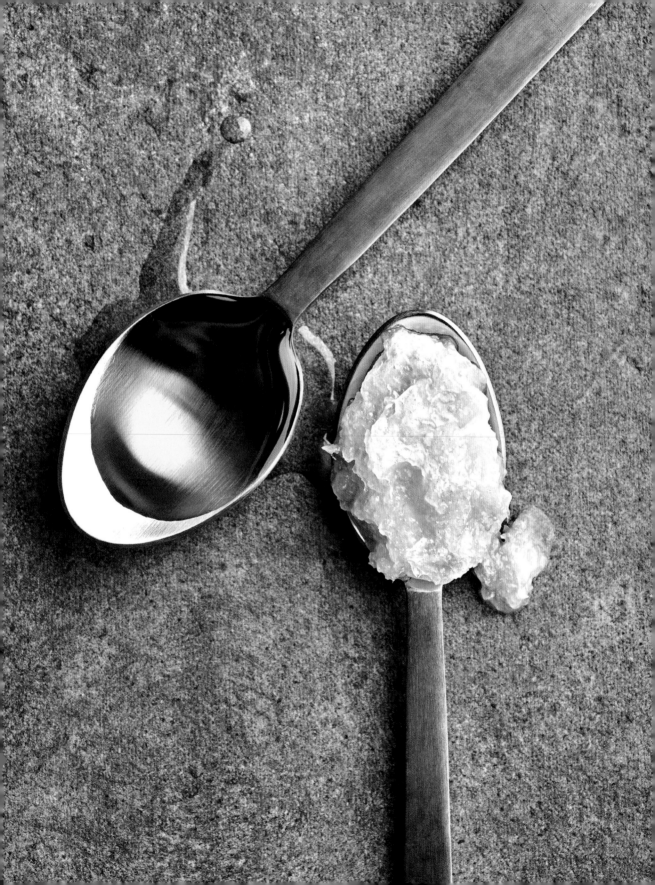

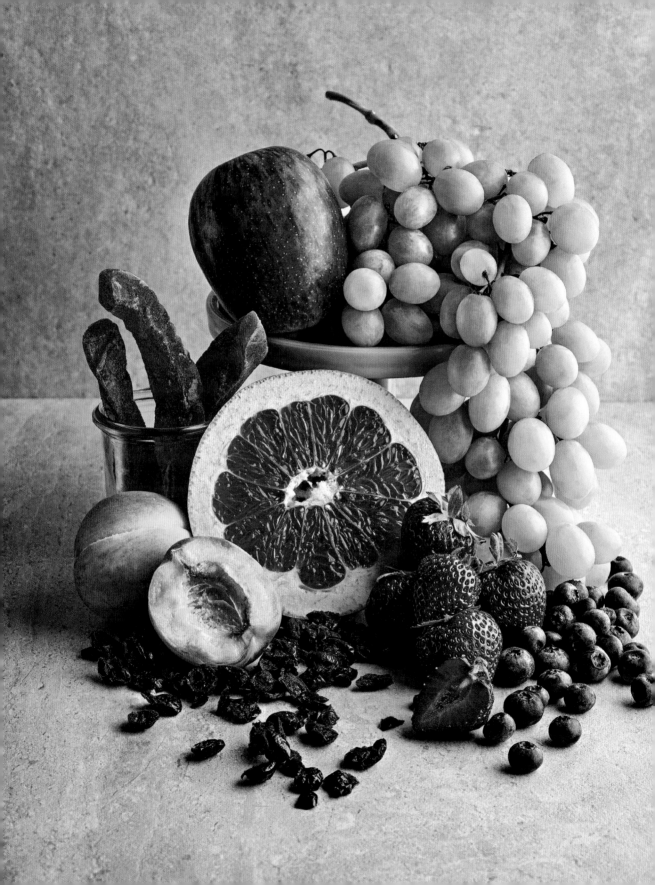

ACT 2 FOODS

These are our eating plan's costars: high-fiber plant foods that play a crucial supporting role. That's because when dietary fat meets dietary fiber, you've got a great duo for shaping your body and boosting weight loss, if that's your goal.

The Ballerina Body way of eating is particularly high in a great fiber source—vegetables, which are especially powerful when it comes to losing and managing weight. But you can also get the fiber you need from eating fruits, nuts, beans, and whole grains. I incorporate all of these food types daily, from my snacks of bananas, dried fruit, and nuts that keep me energized during class, rehearsals, and performances, to the quinoa or lentils that I'll have as an accompaniment at lunch or dinner.

Fibrous Vegetables

Artichokes	Cucumber	Onions	Summer squash
Arugula	Dandelion greens	Parsley	Swiss chard
Asparagus	Eggplant	Pea pods	Tomatoes
Beet greens	Endive	Peppers, all types	Turnip greens
Bok choy	Garlic	Radishes	Water chestnuts
Broccoli	Green beans	Scallions/green	Watercress
Broccoli rabe	Jicama	onions	Zucchini
Brussels sprouts	Kale	Spaghetti squash	
Cabbage, all types	Lettuce, all types	Spinach	
Cauliflower	Mushrooms, all types	Sprouts (alfalfa,	
Celery	Mustard greens	broccoli, mung,	
Collard greens	Okra	and so forth)	

Nutritional benefits: Besides helping to control weight and being loaded with fiber, vegetables are also full of vitamins, minerals, and phytochemicals, from cancer-fighting lycopene in tomatoes to the alphabet soup of vitamins—A, C, K—offered by various greens, to iron- and calcium-rich onions.

Prep tips: You can enjoy the crunch and convenience of eating your veggies raw, though contrary to some beliefs, they're not necessarily more nutritious than their cooked counterparts. In fact, if you steam, grill, lightly cook, or roast your vegetables, you may get an even bigger burst of disease-combating compounds, including lycopene from tomatoes and beta-carotene from carrots.

If you're not buying organically grown vegetables, be sure to carefully wash your foods to get rid of pesticide and other chemical residues.

How to shop: I think fresh is best.

Serving size: You may eat liberally from this list.

Fruits

I've got a sweet tooth, and no doubt so do many of you. Lately I've been loving peanut butter cookies, but fruit is a far better way to satisfy those sweet cravings and bolster your health at the same time. At the start of my day, right after ballet class and before I launch into seven hours of rehearsals, I'll grab a piece of fruit for an energy boost and something refreshing to nibble on.

A really interesting study in the Society for Public Health Education's publication found that those who kept fruit on their kitchen counter and made sure there wasn't candy or soda sitting nearby actually tended to be slimmer. So keep your fruit bowl stocked and in plain sight.

Apples	Cherries	Melon, all varieties	Tangerines
Apricots	Dried fruit (all	Nectarines	Watermelon
Bananas	types—as long	Oranges	
Berries	as they are	Papayas	
Blackberries	unsweetened)	Peaches	
Blueberries	Grapefruit	Pears	
Cranberries	Grapes	Pineapple	
Raspberries	Guava	Plums	
Strawberries	Mango	Tangelos	

Nutritional benefits: Fruits are a potpourri of vitamins, phytochemicals, and fiber that leave you feeling full as well as enhance your health.

Prep tips: Grab, rinse, and eat. Or, chop up your favorites and add to a salad.

How to shop: First—fresh or frozen? Again, stick to what's fresh. Try to pick the brightest, most colorful fruits from the produce section—the brighter the color, the higher the nutrient levels.

Dried fruits are also a healthy option. They're another one of my preferred snacks and make for a great companion to nuts. In fact, when they're eaten together, they're even more powerful, potentially lowering your risk for diabetes and cardiovascular disease. But be mindful: Dried fruit can be higher in sugars and calories than fresh, so watch how much you eat.

Next up—organics: to buy or not to buy? Nowadays most groceries have an organic food section. That means the meats, vegetables, and dairy products have been grown or raised with natural fertilizers and in adherence to other practices that preserve the environment.

If foods are labeled organic, they must meet standards set by the U.S. Department of Agriculture. The jury is still out on whether organic products are healthier than other foods, and they can add up to a more expensive grocery tab. But if you are concerned about the environment or want to limit the pesticide residue or additives you consume (particularly if you will be eating the fruit's skin), organic might be your best option.

Serving size: 1 piece whole fruit (apricots, peaches, etc.); 1 cup fresh berries, melon chunks (cantaloupe, honeydew, watermelon, and similar), tropical fruit chunks (pineapple, mango, papaya, and similar), grapes, or cherries; ¼ cup dried fruits. Have 2 servings of fruit daily.

Fibrous Starches

Starchy foods are complex carbohydrates, which means they're made of numerous sugar units bonded together. Starch occurs naturally in certain vegetables, grains, and cooked dry beans and peas—all high-fiber foods. Although this plan is higher in fat than some other meal plans, I do fit in starchy carbs—though in limited amounts.

Beans and Legumes

Black beans	Cranberry beans	Lima beans	Pinto beans
Chickpeas	Kidney beans	Navy beans	White beans
(garbanzos)	Lentils	Pink beans	

Nutritional benefits: Beans are full of fiber, potassium, and protein. They help to keep bad cholesterol in check, to keep your heart beating strong, and they have a powerful combination of chemicals that may lower your risk of cancer.

Prep tips: Beans are great in soups and stews, or you can season them with spices and a little onion and enjoy.

How to store: Put dried beans inside jars or plastic containers with a lid, then shelve them in a cool space.

Serving size: ½ cup cooked beans or legumes.

Starchy Vegetables

Beets	Parsnips	Turnips	Winter squashes
Carrots	Peas	Sweet potatoes	(such as butter-
Corn	Potatoes		nut and acorn)

Nutritional benefits: A mix of these starchy veggies can be a boon to your overall health, whether it's antioxidant-rich carrots that may help protect against certain forms of cancer, or turnips, overflowing with potassium, which help to regulate blood pressure and cholesterol.

Prep tips: You can mash them, toss them in soups, or steam and serve them as a side.

How to shop: The general rule is the more vibrant the color, the fresher the vegetable. Also make sure there is no obvious bruising or splintering of the skin.

Serving size: ½ cup starchy vegetables.

Whole Grains

These are whole grains as well as sprouted bread, muffins, and bagels.

Note: An asterisk in the list will let you know which grains are gluten-free.

Amaranth*	Instant or	Quinoa*	Whole-grain bread
Bran	quick-cooking	Sprouted bread	(100 percent
Brown rice*	oatmeal	Steel-cut oats	whole-grain)
Buckwheat*	Millet*	White rice*	Wild rice*
Couscous	Pearled barley		

Nutritional benefits: Bursting with fiber, whole grains can strengthen your heart by reducing your blood pressure and bad cholesterol. Adding whole grains to your menu can also help control blood glucose and keep you from becoming constipated.

Prep tips: You can boil a cup of oats for a turbocharging breakfast, fill out your lunch with a hearty side of couscous or brown rice, or simmer quinoa with seafood for a mouth-watering dinner.

How to shop: Read the ingredients. "Whole" should be at the top of the list. If it isn't, there's a strong chance that whole grains make up only a small portion of whatever food you are buying.

Serving size: ½ cup grains, cereals, rice, pasta; 2 slices sprouted or whole-grain bread; 1 muffin; 1 whole wheat bagel. Have only 1 serving of any starchy food daily (including starchy vegetables).

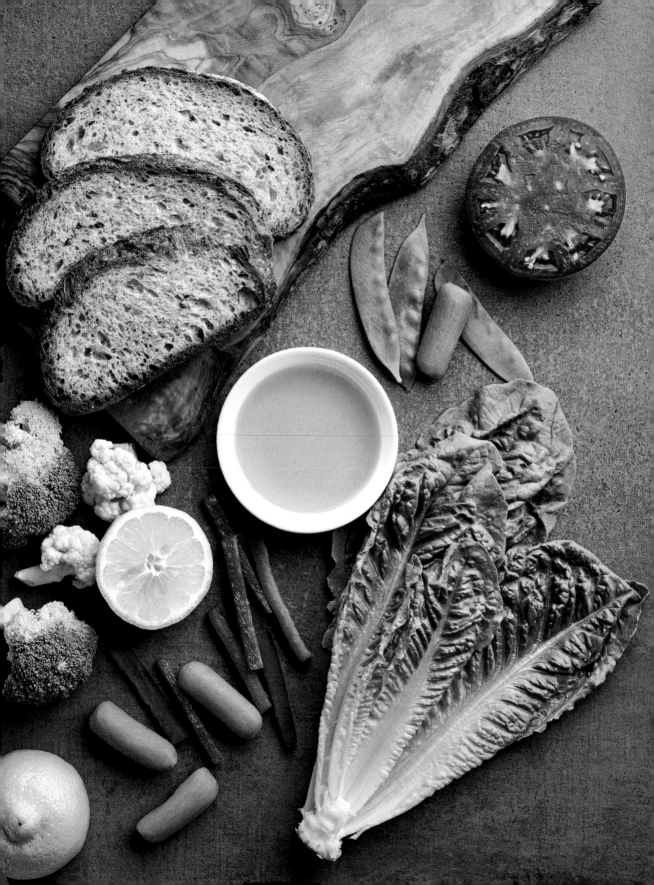

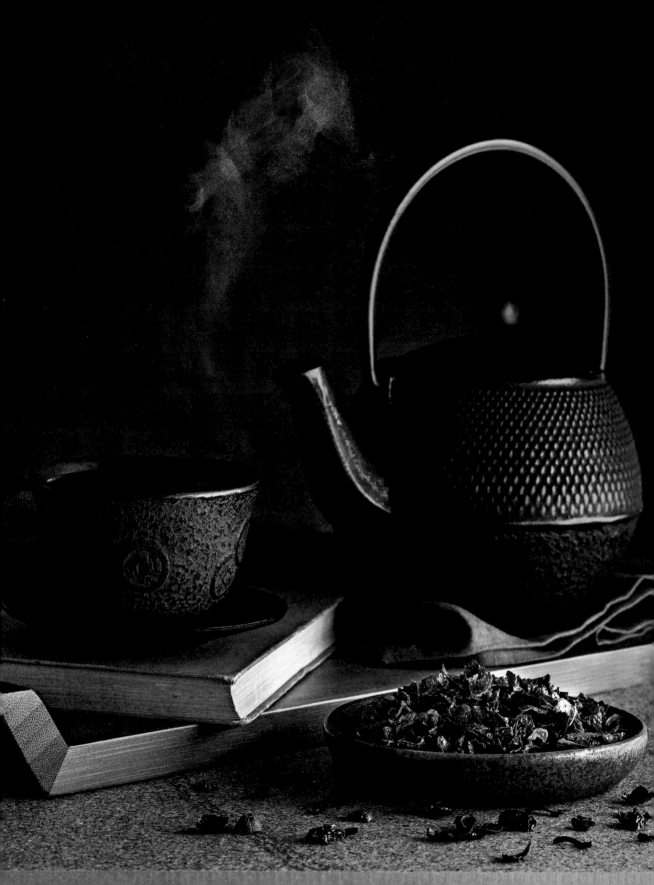

Extras to Choose in Moderation

All-fruit jams

Barbecue sauce (low-sugar)

Dry wines such as Prosecco

Herbs and spices, all types

Horseradish

Hot sauces

Lemon juice

Lime juice

Mayonnaise (fat-free or low-fat)

Mustard, all types

Natural sweeteners (stevia, honey)

Nonstick vegetable sprays

No-sugar-added pasta or marinara sauce

Nut-based milks (almond, cashew, and coconut milks)

Reduced-sugar ketchup

Salad dressings (Homemade is best: Whisk together 2 parts vinegar to 1 part extra-virgin olive oil. Add herbs such as basil, oregano, garlic powder, and a little salt and pepper to taste, and mix well.)

Salsa

Soy sauce (reduced-sodium)

Vinegars

Have a Cup of Tea

Tea has been a part of ritual and ceremony for centuries. And not only is sipping a cup soothing and warming to the body, but many herbal varieties have medicinal properties as well.

Here are some teas to consider.

- Hibiscus and rose-hip teas, which are reported to strengthen the immune system and prevent high blood pressure
- Lemongrass and milk-thistle teas, which aid in digestion and detoxification
- Ginger tea, which eases stomach troubles and colds
- Blueberry leaf tea to help regulate blood sugar
- Green tea for its antioxidant properties
- Fennel tea for gas and bloating
- Chamomile and lavender tea to assist in relaxation and sleep

HOW TO BREW

- Tea can be prepared from bags or loose leaves, with boiling water poured over the tea leaves or bags. It can be enjoyed hot or cold. If you choose bottled or canned teas, avoid those with added sugar.
- Enjoy as much herbal tea as you like.
- A drink of hot water and lemon when you wake up can be a refreshing and welcome way to start the day.

BALLERINA BODY EATING GUIDELINES

- Try to stick with the foods that are listed.
- At breakfast, lunch, and dinner, always include at least one food from the Act 1 list. For lunch and dinner you'll also choose an option from the Act 2 menu.
- Don't skip meals. Not only can skipping meals cause you to miss nutrients important for your health and performance, but it can also lead to overeating. You become so hungry that "anything goes" and all your good intentions can fly out the window. Oftentimes you end up eating the first thing you can grab, which may not be very nutritious.
- Do not stuff yourself or otherwise get to the point of discomfort at the end of a meal. Eat until you're satisfied; it's okay to leave food on your plate.
- Avoid problem foods. These include liquid calories (sodas), sweets, any food containing added sugar, processed packaged food, junk food, fast food, white flour, white bread, artificial sweeteners, and the oils that fall in the omega-6 family, such as soybean, cottonseed, sunflower, corn, and canola. There's nothing wrong with an occasional cheat like a muffin or a cheese biscuit. But do it sparingly. You don't want to undo all your hard work by going overboard at a single meal.
- Try to eat a variety of foods to make sure you're getting the nutrients that you need and to keep your meals interesting.
- Stay hydrated, since water is vital to keeping your muscles healthy and to burning fat. Drink eight to ten 8-ounce glasses of pure water daily.
- Enjoy two snacks every day.

How to Snack Healthily

Carry Your Own: It's a smart idea to carry your own small bites so you don't wind up grabbing whatever's available—and often not so healthy—when hunger pangs hit.

Load Up on Nuts and Fruit: They're easy to tuck inside your pocket or bag, really good for you, and filling enough that when you're at the movies, you won't be tempted to buy a bunch of candy at the concession counter. Along with my nuts, I love dried fruit and bananas. And for a nice blend of salty and sweet, I'll sometimes pack a bag of grapes along with lightly salted air-popped popcorn.

Down the Water: You can't go wrong with water. It's a sugar-free elixir that your body can't live without, and it also helps quell your hunger. Often when we think we want to eat, we're really craving water instead.

How to Eat While on the Road

Pack Your Nutrition: Airports are starting to feature healthier options than the traditional burgers and pizza, but to be safe—and save a few dollars while I'm at it—I like to take along packaged food that I can rely on to give my body what it needs, especially if I'm heading overseas. I usually carry packets of plain oatmeal, packaged tuna, whole wheat crackers, and nuts.

How to Dine Out and Eat Well

Choose Wisely: It can be tough to stay committed to eating healthy when you're surrounded by other diners ordering delicious-looking sweets and fried foods. But you can summon the willpower to stick to your eating plan and still feel satisfied. Even if I'm eating at one of my guilty pleasures, Red Lobster, I like to go with options that don't have a ton of empty calories added to them. For instance, I'll order the crab legs and a garden salad. Go for clean—a piece of fish that isn't breaded or fried, a salad or vegetable, and quinoa, lentils, or couscous instead of rice.

My Perfect Day

I'd have a muffin or bagel slathered with scallion cream cheese, which I'd wash down with an iced coffee. During the day, I'd nibble on cashews and macadamia nuts along with some dried pineapple and a few grapes. Lunch would be a delicious spinach salad topped with pecans, goat cheese, dried cranberries, and a light vinaigrette. Dinner would be a piece of grilled salmon, with roasted onions, carrots, and butternut squash seasoned with rosemary, garlic, and a bit of salt and pepper. Since I would have been conscientious all day, hydrating constantly with water, I'd have a glass of Prosecco and maybe a peanut butter cookie for dessert!

Power Booster

"My Perfect Day" menu would be my ideal when it comes to taste alone, but when I want a delicious meal that's also going to give me a burst of energy to power me through my workout, these are the foods I go for: oatmeal for breakfast, a Mediterranean Wrap (page 169) for lunch, and Coconut Quinoa and Lentil Curry (page 185) for dinner.

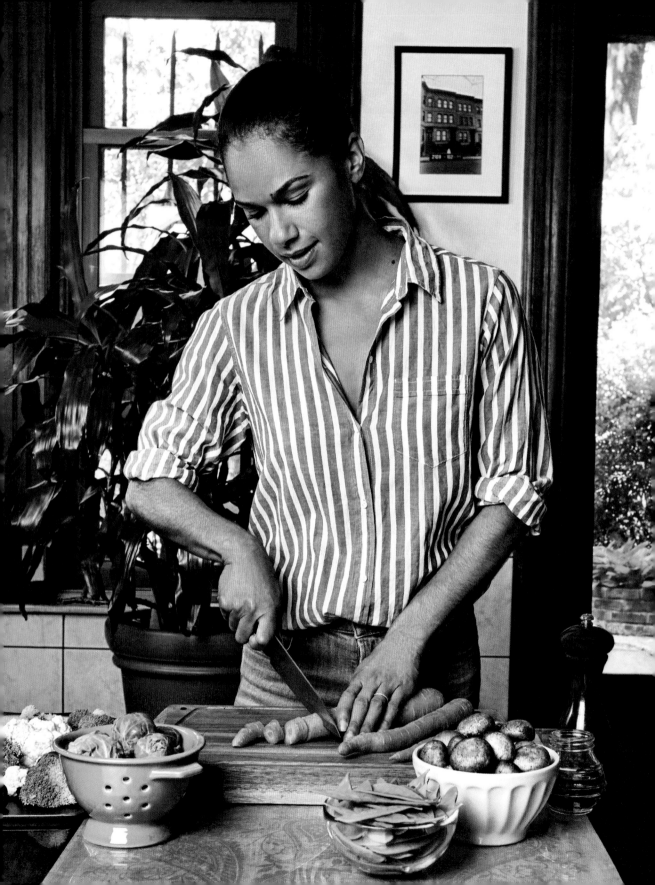

Chapter 9

MEAL CHOREOGRAPHY

H ere's my blueprint for how you can structure your meals, something I call meal choreography. Like a ballet and our workout routine, which take a medley of basic steps and build from there in combination and complexity, you'll be able to mix and match a variety of foods to make sure you enjoy what you're eating and your taste buds don't get bored. Eating a range of foods also ensures that you get all the nutrients you need for optimal health and fat burning without filling up on foods that may not be as helpful.

You'll also be eating for energy. Each meal in this plan has a combination of protein, carbohydrates, and fat to optimize your endurance, help make your thinking laser sharp, maximize your digestive function, and keep cravings at bay. And to make your meal planning a little simpler, I've included suggestions covering twenty-one days. You can find all the recipes in Chapter 10 (page 145).

For Breakfast

Every day, choose one of these seven options:

1. Bran Muffin (**page 152**) with High-Fiber Blender Jam (optional; **page 191**), 6 ounces of Greek yogurt, coffee or tea

2. Ballerina Smoothie (**page 203**), coffee or tea

3. Whole-grain bagel with High-Fiber Blender Jam (**page 191**), a piece of fresh fruit, coffee or tea

4. Whole-grain toast, a cooked egg, a piece of fresh fruit, coffee or tea

5. Granola (**page 148**) with almond milk, coffee or tea

6. Oatmeal with Brown Sugar (**page 147**), coffee or tea

7. Egg White Frittata (**page 151**), coffee or tea

For Lunch

Choose Act 1 foods, plus Act 2 vegetables (preferably raw). Example: tuna atop a bed of raw salad veggies, drizzled with salad dressing.

For Dinner

Choose Act 1 foods, plus Act 2 vegetables and a starchy plant food. Example: grilled fish, green beans, and a serving of brown rice.

For Snacks

Choose two daily:

A piece, or handful, of fresh fruit (any kind; my favorites are grapes, blueberries, dried mango, and banana)

A handful of dried fruit and a handful of nuts (my favorites are pistachios, almonds, and cashews)

A hard-boiled egg

A serving of cheese, including cottage cheese

1 cup yogurt

A handful of veggie sticks or kale chips

Sushi (3 to 4 pieces)

Seafood: oysters (2 or 3 large), shrimp (5 or 6), clams (6 or 7), and any food you can sample at a raw bar

21-DAY BALLERINA BODY MEAL PLAN

Week 1

Day 1

BREAKFAST

Whole-grain bagel with 1 tablespoon *High-Fiber Blender Jam* (page 191)

1 piece of fruit

Coffee or tea

SNACK

1 banana

LUNCH

Large spinach salad topped with pecans, 2 to 3 slices of avocado, ⅓ cup crumbled goat cheese, and dried cranberries, drizzled with a vinaigrette dressing (page 170)

SNACK

1 handful of macadamia nuts

DINNER

Citrus Salmon (page 177)

Roasted Vegetables (page 160)

1 glass of dry white wine or Prosecco (optional)

Day 2

BREAKFAST

Bran Muffin (page 152)

6 ounces Greek yogurt

1 tablespoon *High-Fiber Blender Jam* (page 191), spread on your muffin or stirred into your yogurt

Coffee or tea

SNACK

1 handful of *Fruit and Nut Medley* (page 202)

LUNCH

Colorful Shrimp Caesar Salad (page 166)

SNACK

4 *Misty and Makeda's Banana Oatmeal Cookies* (page 201)

DINNER

Baked whitefish

½ cup brown rice

Roasted Vegetables (page 160)

Day 3

BREAKFAST

Ballerina Smoothie (page 203)

Coffee or tea

SNACK

1 medium apple

LUNCH

Ultimate Veggie Burger (page 189)

SNACK

Kale Chips (page 198)

DINNER

Grilled tofu

Mashed Butternut Squash (page 178)

Day 4

BREAKFAST

Whole-grain toast

1 cooked egg (poached, hard-boiled, soft-boiled, or scrambled)

1 piece of fruit

Coffee or tea

SNACK

¼ cup cottage cheese with cut-up raw vegetables (cucumbers, baby carrots, broccoli, and so forth, for dipping)

LUNCH

Mediterranean Wraps with Garden Pesto (page 169)

SNACK

Yummus and Veggies (page 197)

DINNER

Black Bean Soup with Lime Shrimp (page 155)

Day 5

BREAKFAST

Granola (page 148) with almond milk

Coffee or tea

SNACK

2 ounces tofu

4 whole wheat crackers

LUNCH

Loaded Mock Potato Soup (page 194)

SNACK

Carrot Juice (page 203)

DINNER

Flounder with Sautéed Kale (page 173)

Day 6

BREAKFAST

Oatmeal with Brown Sugar (page 147)

Coffee or tea

SNACK

1 orange

LUNCH

Sandwich made with 1 mini whole wheat pita, 4 ounces tofu or sliced cheese, ½ roasted
pepper, 1 tablespoon light mayonnaise, mustard, and lettuce

SNACK

1 handful of *Fruit and Nut Medley* (page 202)

DINNER

Sushi and seaweed salad (at an Asian restaurant), or if you're eating at home, 4 ounces of
baked whitefish and *Roasted Vegetables* (page 160)

Day 7

BREAKFAST

Egg White Frittata (page 151)

Coffee or tea

SNACK

Yummus and Veggies (page 197)

LUNCH

Spinach and Goat Cheese Salad (page 159)

SNACK

1 cup cantaloupe chunks or other melon in season

DINNER

Quick Salsa Chili (page 179)

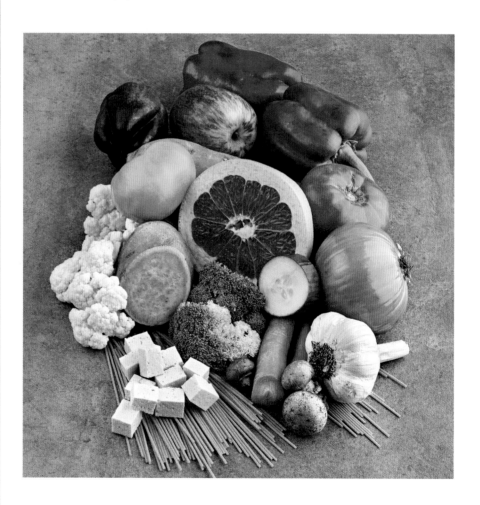

GROCERY LIST: Staples to Have on Hand for All 3 Weeks

Spices and Flavorings

Cardamom
Chili powder
Cinnamon
Crushed red pepper
Cumin
Curry powder
Dried Italian spices
    (typically a medley of
    basil, oregano, rose-
    mary, onion powder,
    and garlic powder)

Fish sauce
Ginger
Paprika
Pepper
Salts, including sea salt
    and kosher salt
Thai red curry
    paste
Turmeric
Vanilla extract
White pepper, ground

Baking Ingredients

Baking soda
Coconut flour
Cornstarch

Raw cacao powder
Unsweetened coconut
    flakes

Grains

Bran
Brown rice
Oatmeal packets
    (10-count package)

Panko bread crumbs
Quinoa, red and white
Whole wheat crackers
    (1 box)

Nuts and Seeds

Almonds
Cashews
Flaxseeds
Hemp seeds

Macadamia nuts
Pecans
Sesame seeds
Walnuts

Sweetening Agents

Agave syrup
Brown sugar

Honey
Maple syrup

Condiments

Apple cider vinegar
Balsamic vinegar
Hot sauce
Lemon juice (bottled)
Low-sodium soy sauce

Reduced-sugar ketchup
Red wine vinegar
White cooking wine
White wine vinegar

Fats, Oils, and Salad Dressings

Almond butter
Caesar Dressing
    (homemade,
    page 171)
Coconut oil
Italian Dressing (home-
    made, page 170)
Light mayonnaise
Mustard
Extra-virgin olive oil

Raspberry Vinaigrette
    (homemade,
    page 171)
Sesame oil
Tahini
Vegetable cooking
    spray
Vinaigrette (homemade,
    page 170)

Other

Coffee
Nondairy milk
Tea

Prosecco
    (1 bottle, optional)

GROCERY LIST FOR WEEK 1

Vegetables

Arugula (16-ounce package)

Assortment of raw veggies: cucumbers, baby carrots, broccoli, cauliflower

Avocado

Broccoli (1 head)

Brussels sprouts (2 to 3 packages, 20 ounces each)

Butternut squash (1)

Carrots (2 to 3 small bags)

Cauliflower (2 to 3 heads)

Chives (1 package)

Flat-leaf parsley (1 bunch)

Basil (3 packages, 1.25 ounces each)

Rosemary (1 package)

Thyme (1 package)

Garlic (2 bulbs)

Green bell pepper (1)

Kale (3 to 4 packages, 16 ounces each)

Lettuce (1 head)

Mushrooms (2 to 3)

Onions, white and yellow (6 to 7)

Peas, fresh (1 large bag)

Red bell pepper (2)

Red onion (1)

Romaine lettuce (2 heads)

Roma tomatoes (2)

Scallions (1 bunch)

Snow peas (1 bag)

Spinach (2 packages, about 16 ounces each)

Baby spinach (2 packages, 16 ounces each)

Fruits

Apples (3 to 4)

Applesauce, unsweetened, 24-ounce jar

Bananas (3)

Berries (1 small carton), any type

Cantaloupe

1 package each dried apricots, dried cherries, dried cranberries, pitted prunes, dried Mission figs, chopped dates, Medjool dates, and raisins

Lemons (1)

Limes (2)

Orange (1)

Other fruits as desired for snacking

Fruit Juice

Orange juice (carton)

Prune juice (bottled)

Breads and Cereal

Rolled oats (42-ounce carton)

Whole-grain bagels (1)

Whole wheat hamburger rolls (1 package)

Loaf of whole-grain bread

Low-carb flour tortillas (1 package)

Whole wheat pita bread (1 package)

Nuts and Seeds

1 package each (25 ounces): almonds, cashews, dates, macadamia nuts, pecans, and walnuts

Seafood

Flounder (2 fillets, 4 to 5 ounces each)

Salmon (1 pound)

Shrimp (40)

Whitefish (2 fillets, 4 ounces each)

Dairy

Cottage cheese (small curd, 16 ounces)

Goat cheese

Eggs (2 cartons)

Mozzarella cheese (8 ounces fresh)

Greek yogurt (12 ounces)

Parmesan cheese, grated

Small carton of heavy cream

Small carton of half-and-half

Swiss cheese, shredded

Other

Tofu (3 packages)

Black beans (4 cans, 15 ounces each)

Chocolate chips (1 bag, 12 ounces)

Kidney beans (1 can, 15 ounces)

Chunky salsa (2 jars)

Diced fire-roasted tomatoes (1 can, 14 ounces)

Roasted red peppers (1 jar, 16 ounces)

Tomato sauce (1 can, 15 ounces)

Low-sodium vegetable broth (5 cartons, 32 ounces each)

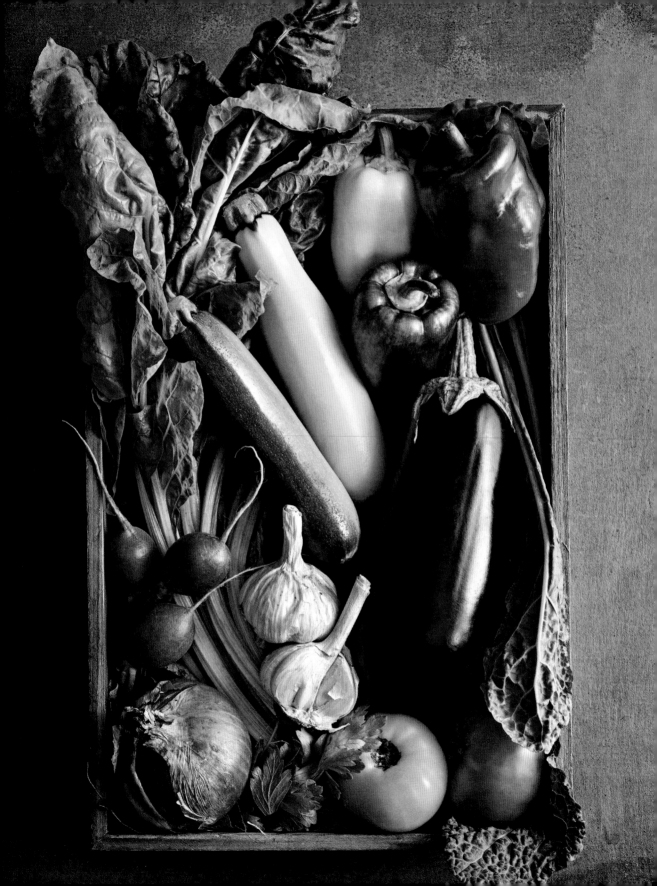

Week 2

Day 8

BREAKFAST

Bran Muffin (page 152)

6 ounces Greek yogurt

1 tablespoon *High-Fiber Blender Jam* (page 191), spread on your muffin or stirred into your
yogurt

Coffee or tea

SNACK

1 cup fresh strawberries, sliced and topped with 2 tablespoons Greek yogurt sweetened
with 1 teaspoon honey

LUNCH

Tuna Niçoise Salad (page 165)

SNACK

1 *Misty's Raw Barre* (page 192)

DINNER

Flounder with Sautéed Kale (page 173)

Day 9

BREAKFAST

Whole-grain bagel with 1 tablespoon *High-Fiber Blender Jam* (page 191)

1 piece of fruit

Coffee or tea

SNACK

1 apple

LUNCH

Tuna Niçoise Salad (page 165)

SNACK

Kale Chips (page 198)

DINNER

Coconut Quinoa and Lentil Curry (page 185)

Day 10

BREAKFAST

Bran Muffin (page 152)

6 ounces Greek yogurt

1 tablespoon *High-Fiber Blender Jam* (page 191), spread on your muffin or stirred into your
 yogurt

Coffee or tea

SNACK

1 medium orange

LUNCH

Mediterranean Wraps with Garden Pesto (page 169)

SNACK

1 handful of *Fruit and Nut Medley* (page 202)

DINNER

Tofu-Veggie Stir-Fry (page 184)

Day 11

BREAKFAST

Ballerina Smoothie (page 203)

Coffee or tea

SNACK

1 *Misty's Raw Barre* (page 192)

LUNCH

Colorful Shrimp Caesar Salad (page 166)

SNACK

1 apple

DINNER

Zoodles Primavera (page 183)

Day 12

BREAKFAST

Granola (page 148) with almond milk

Coffee or tea

SNACK

1 cup fresh strawberries, sliced and topped with 2 tablespoons Greek yogurt

LUNCH

Spinach and Goat Cheese Salad (page 159)

SNACK

1 *Misty's Raw Barre* (page 192)

DINNER

Citrus Salmon (page 177)

Lentils (page 163)

Day 13

BREAKFAST

Oatmeal with Brown Sugar (page 147)

Coffee or tea

SNACK

1 apple

LUNCH

Colorful Shrimp Caesar Salad (page 166)

SNACK

Carrot Juice (page 203)

DINNER

Moroccan Scallops with Quinoa (page 180)

Day 14

BREAKFAST

Egg White Frittata (page 151)

Coffee or tea

SNACK

¼ cup cottage cheese with cut-up raw vegetables (cucumbers, baby carrots, and broccoli)

LUNCH

Loaded Mock Potato Soup (page 194)

SNACK

1 cup yogurt

DINNER

Coconut Quinoa and Lentil Curry (page 185)

GROCERY LIST FOR WEEK 2

Vegetables

Assortment of fresh stir-fry Asian vegetables: scallions, red pepper (sliced), bok choy, broccoli florets, and so forth

Assortment of raw veggies: cucumbers, baby carrots, broccoli, cauliflower

Avocados (2)

Carrots (2 to 3 small bags)

Cauliflower (1 medium)

Celery (1 bag)

Chives (1 package)

Cilantro (1 package)

Fresh basil (3 packages)

Fresh thyme (1 package)

Fresno chili (2)

Garlic (2 bulbs)

Green beans (4 bundles)

Kale (2 packages)

Kale, baby (2 packages, 16 ounces each)

Leeks (1 bunch)

Lentils, French green, such as du Puy (2 bags, 16 ounces each)

Mushrooms (1 small carton)

New potatoes (8)

Onions (8 to 9)

Red bell peppers (6)

Red onion (1)

Romaine lettuce (4 heads)

Roma tomatoes (6)

Salad greens (3 large packages)

Scallions (1 bunch)

Spinach (2 packages, 16 ounces each)

Baby spinach (3 packages, 16 ounces each)

Zucchini (4)

Fruits

Apples (4)

Berries, any type (1 carton)

1 package each dried apricots, dried cherries, dried cranberries, pitted prunes, dried Mission figs, chopped dates, Medjool dates, and raisins

Lemon (2)

Lime (2)

Mango (2)

Orange (1)

Strawberries (2 cartons)

Other fruits as desired for snacking

Fruit Juice

Coconut water (4 cartons, 16.9 ounces each)

Orange juice (carton)

Prune juice (48 ounces)

Seafood

Flounder (2 fillets, 4 to 5 ounces each)

Salmon (1 fillet)

Sea scallops (1½ pounds)

Shrimp (48)

Tuna, packed in water (8 cans, 3 ounces each)

Breads and Cereals

Low-carb tortillas (4)

Whole-grain bagel (1)

Dairy

Cottage cheese (1 carton, 16 ounces)

Eggs (2 cartons)

Goat cheese

Greek yogurt (32 ounces)

Mozzarella cheese, fresh (1 package, 8 ounces)

Parmesan cheese, grated (1 small bag)

Swiss cheese, shredded (1 small bag)

Additional

Black olives, pitted (1 can, 6 ounces)

Tofu (3 to 4 packages)

Low-sodium vegetable broth (4 cartons, 32 ounces each)

Fresh naan

Tomato paste (1 can, 6 ounces)

Coconut milk (2 cans, 14 ounces each)

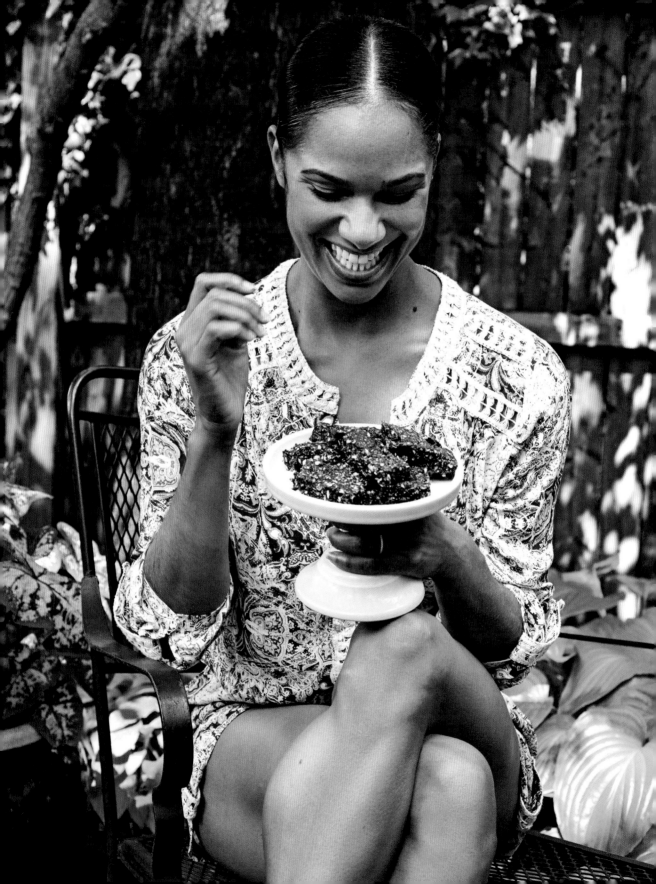

Week 3

Day 15

BREAKFAST

Whole-grain bagel with 1 tablespoon *High-Fiber Blender Jam* (page 191)

1 piece of fruit

Coffee or tea

SNACK

1 cup fresh strawberries, sliced and topped with 2 tablespoons Greek yogurt sweetened
with 1 teaspoon honey

LUNCH

Spinach and Goat Cheese Salad (page 159)

SNACK

1 *Misty's Raw Barre* (page 192)

DINNER

Sushi and seaweed salad (at an Asian restaurant) or, if you're eating at home, *Tuna Niçoise
Salad* (page 165)

Day 16

BREAKFAST

Whole-grain bagel with 1 tablespoon cream cheese

1 piece of fresh fruit

Coffee or tea

SNACK

4 *Misty and Makeda's Banana Oatmeal Cookies* (page 201)

LUNCH

Mediterranean Wraps with Garden Pesto (page 169)

SNACK

1 medium apple

1 handful of almonds

DINNER

Flounder with Sautéed Kale (page 173)

Day 17

BREAKFAST

Ballerina Smoothie (page 203)

Coffee or tea

SNACK

1 medium orange

LUNCH

2 to 3 cups arugula topped with ½ cup halved grape tomatoes and 4 fresh mozzarella
cheese balls and drizzled with *Italian Dressing* (page 170)

SNACK

Yummus and Veggies (page 197)

DINNER

Ultimate Veggie Burger (page 189)

Sweet Potato Fries (page 195)

Day 18

BREAKFAST

Bran Muffin (page 152)

6 ounces Greek yogurt

1 tablespoon *High-Fiber Blender Jam* (page 191), spread on your muffin or stirred into your
yogurt

Coffee or tea

SNACK

1 cup grapes

1 handful of almonds

LUNCH

Tuna Niçoise Salad (page 165)

SNACK

Fruit and Nut Medley (page 202)

DINNER

Loaded Mock Potato Soup (page 194)

Day 19

BREAKFAST

Oatmeal with Brown Sugar (page 147)

Coffee or tea

SNACK

Yummus and Veggies (page 197)

LUNCH

Cobb Salad (at a restaurant), no bacon, ham, or turkey, drizzled with salad dressing, any type

SNACK

1 cup grapes

1 handful of almonds

DINNER

Tofu-Veggie Stir-Fry (page 184)

Day 20

BREAKFAST

Whole-grain toast

1 cooked egg

1 piece of fruit

Coffee or tea

SNACK

1 pear

LUNCH

Brown-bag lunch: 2 slices of whole-grain bread, 2 teaspoons mustard as spread, 2 slices of cheese, ½ cup lettuce, and 2 slices of tomato

SNACK

Carrot Juice (page 203)

DINNER

Sushi and seaweed salad (at an Asian restaurant) or, if you're eating at home, *Ultimate Veggie Burger* (page 189) and *Sweet Potato Fries* (page 195)

Day 21

BREAKFAST

Granola (page 148) with almond milk

Coffee or tea

SNACK

1 handful of almonds or other nuts

LUNCH

Black-bean burrito: 1 tortilla filled with ½ cup mashed or fat-free "refried" black beans, salsa,
2 tablespoons grated reduced-fat cheese, and chopped tomato

SNACK

1 cup melon balls topped with chopped mint

DINNER

Black Bean Soup with Lime Shrimp (page 155)

GROCERY LIST FOR WEEK 3

Vegetables

Assortment of fresh
  stir-fry Asian veg-
  etables: scallions,
  red pepper (sliced),
  bok choy, broccoli
  florets, and
  so forth
Arugula (1 package,
  16 ounces)
Avocados (2)
Carrots (1 bag,
  1 pound)
Cauliflower (1 head)
Chives (1 package)
Basil (6 packages,
  enough for 2 cups
  packed)
Garlic (3 bulbs)
Grape tomatoes
  (1 package)
Green beans
  (2 large bundles,
  enough for 4 cups)

Kale (1 bag, 16 ounces,
  or 2 bundles)
Lettuce (1 small head)
Mint (1 package)
New potatoes (8)
Onion (8 to 9)
Parsley (1 bunch)
Peas, fresh (1 large bag,
  enough for 4 cups)
Red bell pepper (1)
Red onion (1)
Roma tomatoes (6)
Salad greens
  (1 package)
Mixed greens
  (2 packages,
  16 ounces each)
Baby spinach
  (3 packages,
  16 ounces each)
Sweet potatoes
  (4 large)
Tomato (1)

Fruits

Apples (2)
Bananas (2)
Berries, any type
  (1 small carton)
Grapes (1 bunch)
1 package each dried
  apricots, dried cher-
  ries, dried cranber-
  ries, pitted prunes,
  dried Mission figs,
  chopped dates,

Medjool dates, and
  raisins
Melon balls (1 carton)
Lemon (1)
Lime (2)
Orange (1)
Pear (1)
Strawberries (1 carton)
Other fruits as desired
  for snacking

Breads and Cereal

Rolled oats
  (1 carton,
  42 ounces)
Whole-grain bagel (2)

Whole wheat hamburger
  rolls (8)
Low-carb flour tortillas
  (5)

Seafood

Flounder (2 fillets,
  4 to 5 ounces each)
Shrimp (16 jumbo size)

Canned tuna, packed in
  water (8 cans,
  3 ounces each)

Dairy

Eggs (1 carton)
American cheese
  (2 slices)
Cream cheese (1 pack-
  age, 4 ounces)
Goat cheese
Greek yogurt
  (12 ounces)
Mozzarella cheese balls
  (4 fresh)

Mozzarella cheese
  (8 ounces fresh)
Parmesan cheese,
  grated
Reduced-fat cheese (1
  small bag, shredded)
Swiss cheese (1 small
  bag, shredded)
Heavy cream
  (1 small carton)

Additional

Tofu (1 package,
  16 ounces)
Black beans (6 cans,
  15 ounces each)
Fat-free refried black
  beans (1 can,
  15 ounces)

Fire-roasted tomatoes,
  diced (1 can,
  14 ounces)
Black olives, pitted
  (1 can, 6 ounces)
Low-sodium vegetable
  broth (5 cartons,
  32 ounces each)

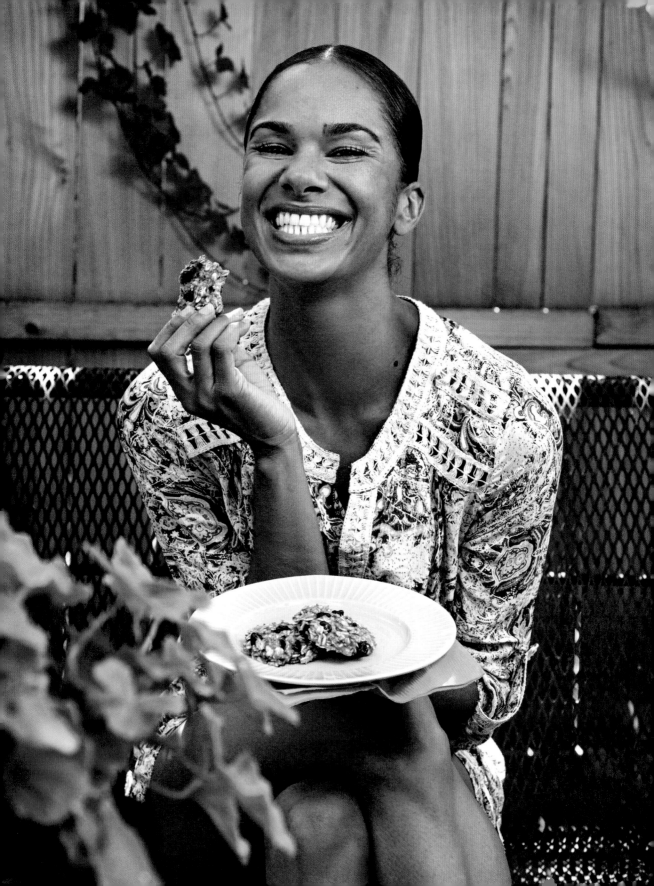

Chapter 10

BALLERINA BODY RECIPES

love to cook. Whether I'm picking out a fresh piece of fish at the supermarket or chopping up vegetables in my kitchen, planning and preparing a meal for myself and the people I love give me a lot of joy. It's all the more special because I realize how essential good nutrition is to having the health and energy we need to accomplish any and every endeavor we want to take on.

I began to experiment in the kitchen out of necessity as I tried to figure out which foods were best for my body. But I soon discovered that cooking was another outlet for my creativity as I improvised a new dish or reinvented an old favorite with a new blend of seasonings and herbs. I also appreciated seeing the reactions of my friends when they enjoyed something I'd whipped up, and the camaraderie of sitting with people I care about, talking, laughing, and savoring a good meal.

I also love to eat! I know that many of us worry that we'll have to sacrifice taste and the pleasure that comes from diving into a luscious plate of food when we're focused on becoming our healthiest selves. But one of the great things about cooking is that you know every ingredient—every pop of spice, every drop of sweetness—that is going into the pot, so you can make your food tasty *and* feel confident that what you're eating is as good for you as it is delicious.

Here, I offer recipes that are diverse enough that you won't get bored, healthy enough to move you closer to your fitness goals, and delectable enough that you won't feel deprived. Because I believe our journey to looking and feeling great shouldn't be blocked by a lot of unnecessary obstacles, I've also tried to make sure that none of these recipes take a ton of time to prepare. Still, you will need to carve a little time out of your day to spend in the kitchen. I hope you'll agree that it's time well spent.

Curtain Raiser

Breakfast is the way we kick-start our day, making sure we are fully energized as we head out the door. On weekdays, I like a bite that gives me a morning jolt, keeping me focused in ballet class and helping me power through my exercises. Typically that means a warm muffin or a steaming cup of oatmeal. But during the weekend, when I have a little more time, I love to blend some homemade juice or whip up a nice frittata. It's an especially delicious way to start the day.

OATMEAL WITH BROWN SUGAR

This is a simple but yummy meal—I make it nearly every morning. You can use plain Quaker oatmeal or any other brand you prefer. I usually add two tablespoons of flaxseed, a second great source of fiber. One of the best things about oatmeal is that on a day when you have a presentation or an exam, a few spoonfuls can help sharpen your memory and concentration. So even when you're in a hurry, warm up a cup and enjoy.

Makes 1 serving

1 packet (single serving) Quaker oatmeal

1 teaspoon brown sugar
2 tablespoons flaxseed

Follow the instructions on the package for making 1 serving of the oatmeal of your choice. Add the brown sugar and flaxseed. Or, if you prefer, you can replace the sugar and flaxseed with a handful of iron-boosting raisins, nuts, or another one of your favorite sources of fiber.

GRANOLA

What's fun about having homemade granola around is all the things you can do with it! A quick breakfast for me would be a handful of granola over Greek yogurt. Or, for a sweet snack that gives you a burst of energy, you can try my granola and peanut butter mix. I started making this when I was about nineteen, and I prepare it often because it's so simple and delicious. Line a bowl with two or three tablespoons of peanut butter, then pour a couple of handfuls of this granola on top. Drizzle in some honey if you want some extra sweetness, then mix it all together and dive in with a spoon. It's like dipping into a bowl of fudge, but instead of a lot of sugar and fat, you're getting a healthy, nutty dose of fiber and protein. A glass of almond milk on the side makes this treat complete.

Makes about 10 servings (10 cups)

3 cups rolled oats (not instant!)

3 tablespoons brown sugar

½ teaspoon ground cinnamon

¼ teaspoon kosher salt

⅓ cup honey

¼ cup extra-virgin olive oil

1 teaspoon vanilla extract

½ cup small-dice dried fruit

½ cup coarsely chopped raw or toasted nuts or seeds

Preheat the oven to 300°F and arrange a rack in the middle.

Place the oats, brown sugar, cinnamon, and salt in a large bowl and stir to combine.

Combine the honey, oil, and vanilla in a small bowl and stir until blended. Pour the honey mixture over the oat mixture and blend until the oats are thoroughly coated.

Spread the mixture in a thin, even layer on a rimmed baking sheet. Bake for 15 minutes, then stir and continue baking until the granola is very light golden brown, 5 to 15 more minutes.

Place the baking sheet on a wire rack and cool the granola to room temperature, about 20 minutes, stirring occasionally. The granola will harden as it cools.

Mix the fruit and nuts or seeds into the granola.

You can store leftovers in an airtight container and keep it in your pantry for later.

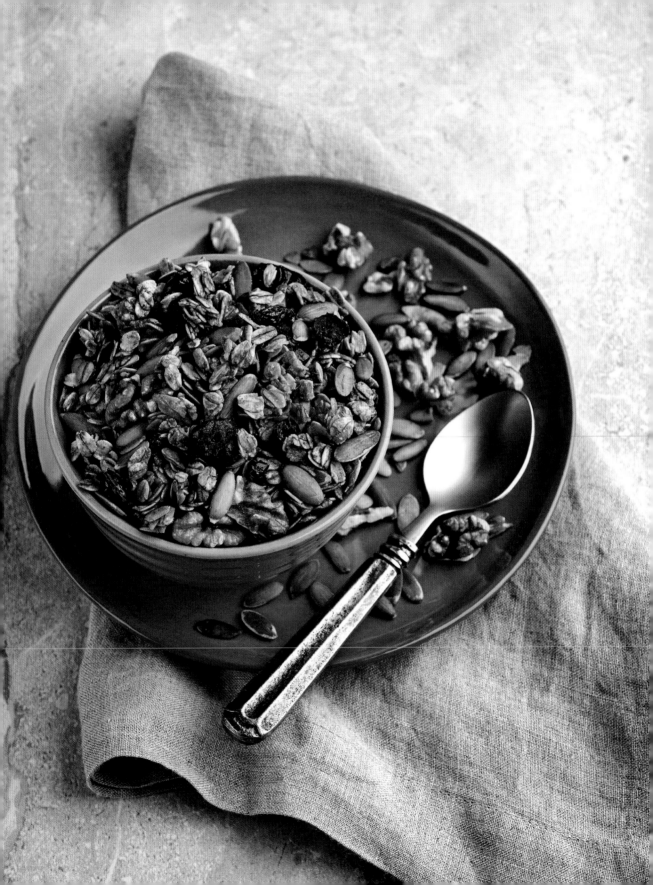

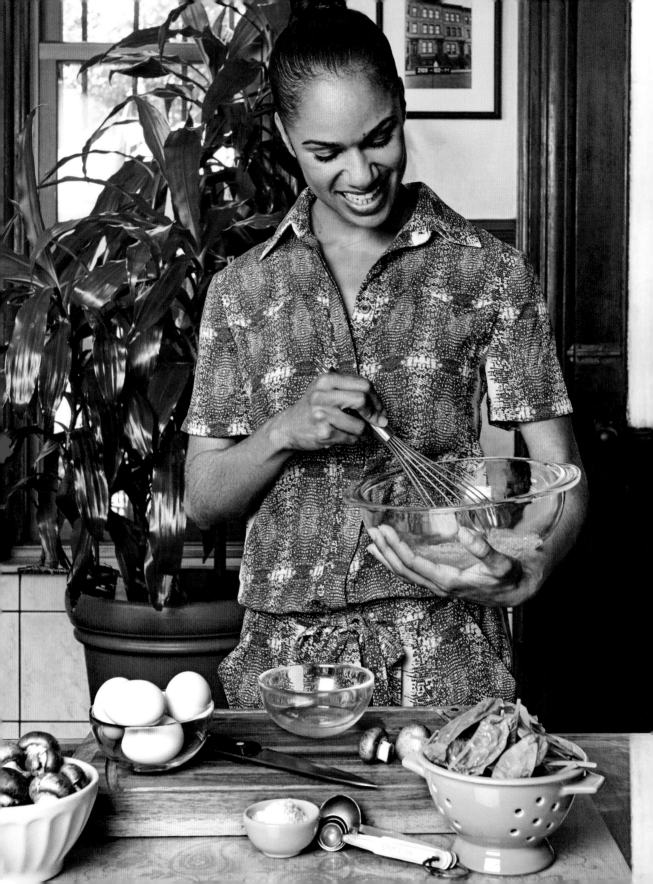

EGG WHITE FRITTATA

When I started seriously dating Olu, this was one of the first dishes I cooked for him. It's quick and super easy to make, which is great on mornings when you are rushing out the door. But the cheese and vegetables turn it into a savory gourmet bite that your guests will think took a lot more time to prepare!

Makes 2 servings

Vegetable cooking spray
2 to 3 mushrooms, sliced
1 handful fresh spinach
1 cup egg whites (8 whites)

Kosher salt
2 tablespoons grated Parmesan
   cheese
Hot sauce (optional)

Preheat the oven or toaster oven to broil.

Spritz a 7-inch oven-safe nonstick frying pan with cooking spray and warm over medium heat.

Add the mushrooms and cook for 2 to 3 minutes, turning once or twice.

Toss in the fresh spinach and cook for 1 to 2 minutes, or until the spinach has wilted.

Whisk the egg whites in a bowl until light and frothy. Add a pinch of kosher salt and add the egg whites to the frying pan.

Sprinkle with 1 tablespoon of the Parmesan.

Let the egg whites cook undisturbed until the edges start to cook through and turn a solid white.

Gently lift the edges of the egg whites and tilt the pan so the uncooked egg white runs under the cooked part. Cook for another minute.

Transfer the frying pan to the oven and broil for 2 to 3 minutes or until the eggs have puffed and cooked through. Remove from the oven and sprinkle with the remaining 1 tablespoon Parmesan cheese. Cut into wedges and serve with hot sauce if desired.

BRAN MUFFINS

Along with oatmeal, muffins are my go-to morning meal. There's something comforting and particularly satisfying about a luscious morning pastry, but the great thing about these particular muffins is that the bran is also really good for you, and the honey and applesauce give the muffins just enough sweetness.

Makes 12 muffins

½ cup coconut flour
¼ cup bran
½ teaspoon baking soda
¼ teaspoon salt
6 eggs

¼ cup coconut oil
½ cup honey
¼ cup unsweetened applesauce
1 teaspoon vanilla extract
Vegetable cooking spray

Preheat the oven to 350°F.

In a small bowl, combine the flour, bran, baking soda, and salt.

In a medium bowl, whisk the eggs. Mix in the oil, honey, applesauce, and vanilla. Add the flour mixture and mix well. Let sit for 5 minutes so that the coconut flour can absorb the liquid.

Spray a 12-cup muffin tin with cooking spray.

Pour the batter into the muffin tins, filling each muffin tin three-quarters full.

Bake for 25 to 30 minutes, or until brown.

Let the muffins cool before serving. Extra muffins can be stored in an airtight container in the refrigerator for up to 7 days.

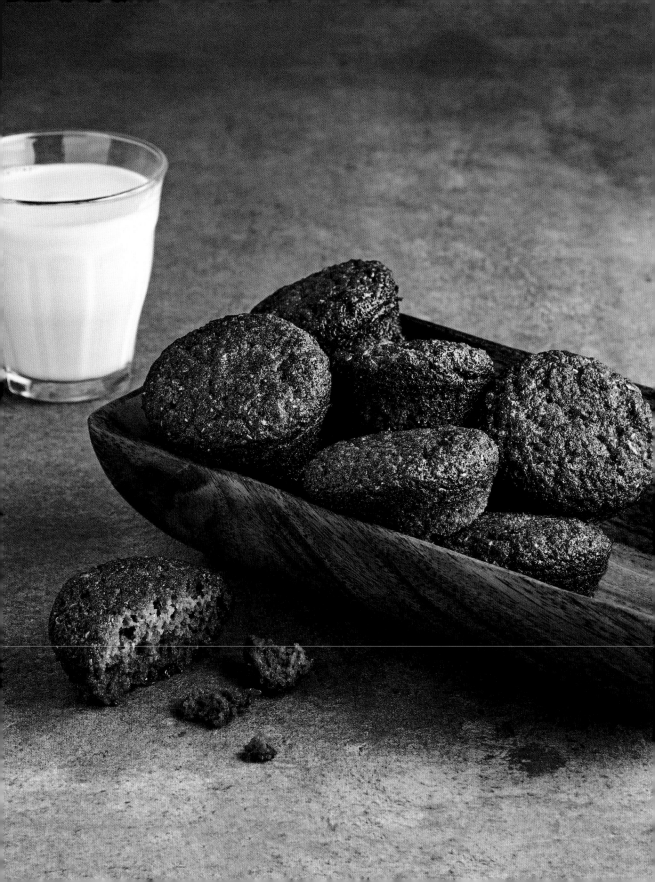

Intermezzo

By lunchtime, not only are you hungry, but you probably need a midday bounce. Since most of us still have hours of work to do, classes to take, and errands to run before we can wrap things up and head home, try to keep lunch light but full of flavor, with ingredients that will give you a burst of energy. I may have a wrap full of veggies and cheese, a rich bowl of soup, or a refreshing plate of sushi.

Whatever's on the menu, try not to skip your midday meal. During a whirlwind of a day, lunch can be a pleasant and energizing interlude.

BLACK BEAN SOUP
WITH LIME SHRIMP

This soup was one of the first recipes I felt really confident cooking. It tastes great and is filling. I learned it from one of the cookbooks written by celebrity chef Rachael Ray, and when I appeared on her show as part of my role with the President's Council on Fitness, Sports and Nutrition, Rachael and I got to make it together. Over the years, I've added my own touches here and there—a little more spice, a little less salt—and used veggie broth instead of chicken.

Makes 4 servings

FOR THE SOUP

2 tablespoons extra-virgin olive oil

1 onion, chopped

3 cloves garlic, chopped

1 teaspoon cumin

2 tablespoons chili powder

Salt and pepper

2 (14-ounce) cans black beans, rinsed and drained

1 (14-ounce) can diced fire-roasted tomatoes

½ cup heavy cream

5 cups low-sodium vegetable broth

Hot sauce

FOR THE SHRIMP

1 clove garlic, chopped

3 tablespoons extra-virgin olive oil

Zest and juice from 2 limes (make zest by scraping the limes against a grater)

½ teaspoon crushed red pepper

¼ cup chopped parsley

Salt

16 jumbo shrimp, peeled, deveined, and butterflied

MAKE THE SOUP

In a soup pot heat the olive oil over medium-high heat. Add the onion, garlic, cumin, chili powder, and salt and pepper to taste. Stir and cook for a few minutes, until the onions become tender.

Add the black beans to the onion mixture. Use a rubber spatula or potato masher to mash half the beans.

Pour in the tomatoes, heavy cream, and vegetable broth. Let the soup come to a boil. Once it's boiling, reduce the heat to a simmer and cook for about 11 minutes, stirring occasionally.

MAKE THE SHRIMP

In a large bowl, combine the garlic with the olive oil, lime zest, crushed red pepper, parsley, and a sprinkle of salt. Add the shrimp to this mixture and toss them until they are coated; remove the shrimp.

Heat a skillet over medium-high heat. Add the shrimp and cook for 2 or 3 minutes. Flip the shrimp, add the lime juice, and cook for another few minutes, until the shrimp are opaque.

Add the hot sauce to the soup and adjust the salt and pepper to your taste. Ladle the soup into 4 bowls and top each with 4 shrimp.

Solo Stars and Nibbles

These are some of my favorite snacks to simply eat by themselves:

- Cottage cheese
- Yogurt
- Veggie stick chips
- Sushi (especially lobster rolls!)
- Nuts such as pistachios, almonds, and cashews
- Any kind of fruit, but particularly grapes, blueberries, dried mango, and bananas
- Seafood—oysters, shrimp, clams, and pretty much any food you can sample at a raw bar

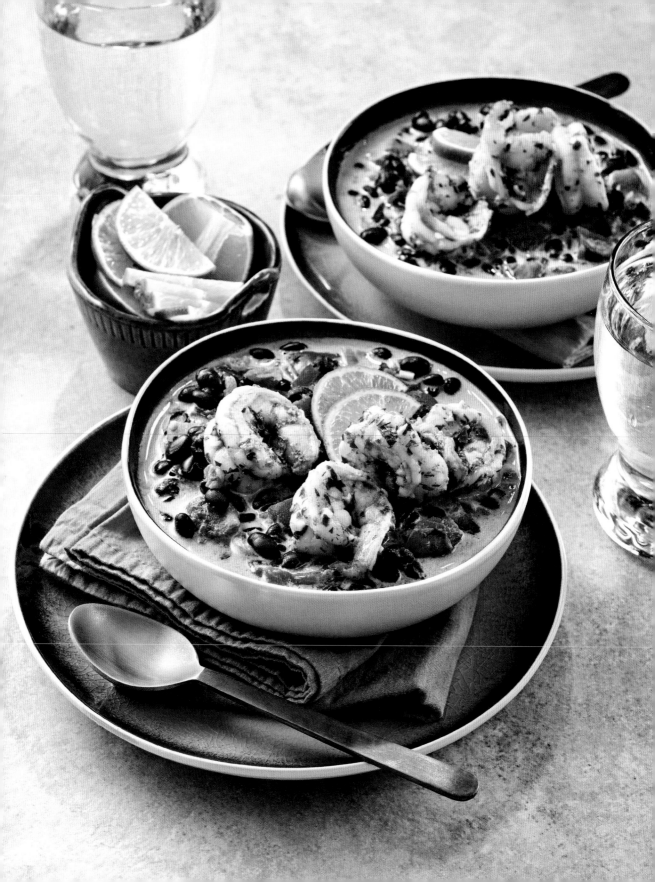

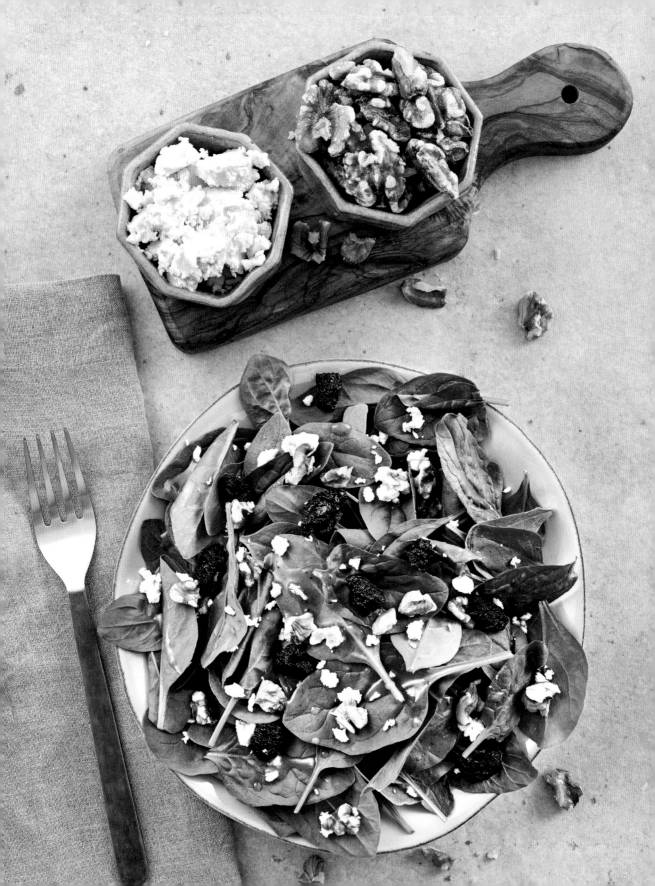

SPINACH AND
GOAT CHEESE SALAD

I love a salad that combines a bunch of my favorite foods, dried fruit, nuts, and a few fluffy dollops of goat cheese. When I eat a plate of this salad, I always feel satisfied but never stuffed. You can have fun mixing and matching the toppings. Maybe toss in some cranberries. Or you can add fish or shrimp and have this salad for dinner.

Makes 4 servings

2 (6-ounce) packages fresh baby spinach, chopped
½ cup dried cherries
½ cup walnuts, chopped

½ cup goat cheese, crumbled
½ red onion, finely chopped
Raspberry Vinaigrette (page 171)

Divide the spinach among 4 plates. Top with the cherries, walnuts, cheese, and onion. Drizzle each plate with 1 tablespoon of homemade raspberry vinaigrette.

ROASTED VEGETABLES

I think roasting really brings out the flavor of vegetables—carrots and snow peas become a bit sweeter, Brussels sprouts taste a bit more nutty. Grab any and every vegetable you love. Some of my favorites are suggested here.

Servings vary:
plan for each person to get a handful, or about a cup, of vegetables

Carrots, peeled

Onion, preferably yellow

Brussels sprouts

Broccoli

Cauliflower

Snow peas

Extra-virgin olive oil

Salt and pepper

Several sprigs thyme

Several sprigs rosemary

Preheat the oven to 375°F.

Cut your vegetables. It's important to make sure all ingredients are pretty much the same size (such as 1-inch chunks) so that they cook evenly.

Place the cut vegetables on large baking sheet. Drizzle with olive oil, season with salt and pepper, and then toss in the thyme and rosemary. Get your hands in there and mix well so that the vegetables are coated with the oil and evenly seasoned.

Place in the oven and roast for 1 hour, or until vegetables are tender and browned slightly. Every 20 minutes, stir and turn the vegetables for even roasting.

Remove from oven. Remove herb sprigs and serve.

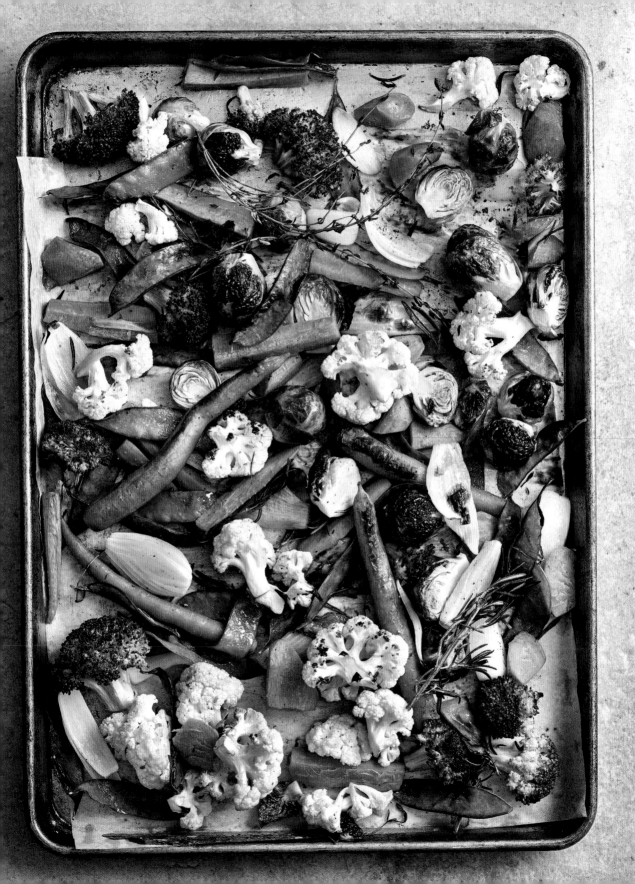

Eat Mindfully

Life moves fast, which is why it's so important to try to be present, in the moment, as often as we can—not just when we're taking a walk, listening to a song that we love, or catching a glimpse of a beautiful sunset as we drive home. It's great to be mindful when we sit down to enjoy a meal as well.

- **Take it slow.** Eating slowly is better for your digestion, allows you to really relish the flavors you're tasting, and can help you realize when you're truly full. When we eat unconsciously we may fill ourselves up more than we should, and we'll feel uncomfortable later—either when we try to go to sleep with a bloated stomach, or when our clothes start to feel tighter than we want them to be.
- **Put the spotlight on your food and friends.** Turn off the television, put your smartphone on vibrate or mute, and turn off your laptop. Focus your attention instead on the meal in front of you, and if you're dining with friends or family, on the conversation you're having. Meals give us a chance to replenish our physical energy and catch up with our loved ones. Moments like those are precious, so let's try to appreciate them.

LENTILS

This recipe was handed down to me by a close friend who is a former ballerina with ABT. She and I both *love* to cook, so about ten years ago, we started a cooking competition. It grew so big that it became a twice-yearly company event. Her lentils are one recipe I'll give her the win for!

Makes 4 servings

½ pound French green lentils
   (such as du Puy)
¼ cup extra-virgin olive oil
2 onions, preferably yellow,
   chopped (about 2 cups)
2 leeks, white and light green parts
   only, chopped (about 2 cups)
1 teaspoon fresh thyme leaves,
   chopped (about 2 sprigs)
2 teaspoons kosher salt
¾ teaspoon freshly ground
   black pepper

4 cloves garlic, minced
   (about 1 tablespoon)
4 stalks celery, chopped
   (about 1½ cups)
3 carrots, chopped (about 1½ cups)
1½ cups low-sodium vegetable
   broth
2 tablespoons tomato paste
2 tablespoons red wine vinegar

Place the lentils in a heatproof bowl and cover with boiling water. Set aside for 15 minutes, then drain and reserve.

Meanwhile, heat the olive oil in a sauté pan over medium heat, add the onions, leeks, thyme, salt, and pepper, and cook for 10 minutes, until the onions are translucent. Add the garlic and cook for 2 more minutes. Add the celery, carrots, vegetable broth, and tomato paste. Add the drained lentils to the pan, then cover and simmer over low heat for 20 minutes (until the lentils are tender). Add the vinegar and season with additional salt and pepper to taste.

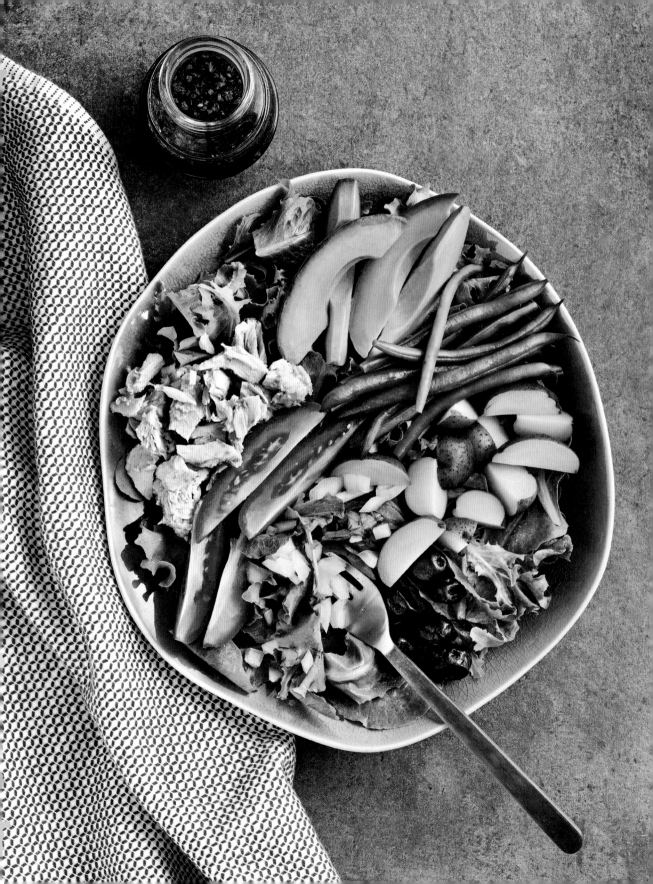

TUNA NIÇOISE SALAD

Tuna is one of those versatile ingredients that's as great by itself as it is in a recipe like this, where it's combined with a bunch of vegetables. You can prepare this the night before, put it in an airtight container, and take it with you to class or work.

Makes 4 servings

6 cups well-packed mixed greens

2 cups green beans, boiled or
    steamed

½ medium onion, diced
    (about ½ cup)

4 new potatoes, boiled and
    quartered

2 Roma tomatoes, cut into wedges

1 ripe avocado, peeled and cut into
    thin pieces

12 black olives, pitted

4 (3-ounce) cans tuna, packed in
    water (12 ounces)

Bottled oil and balsamic vinegar
    salad dressing, or make your own
    by mixing 2 parts extra-virgin
    olive oil to 1 part balsamic
    vinegar

Divide the greens among 4 dinner plates. Top each plate with equal portions of green beans, onion, potatoes, tomatoes, avocado, olives, and tuna. Drizzle about 1 tablespoon of dressing over each salad and serve.

COLORFUL SHRIMP
CAESAR SALAD

A good meal engages so many of our senses. It's not just our taste buds. I love when my kitchen fills with the aromas of whatever I'm cooking, and a beautifully plated meal can resemble a work of art. This salad, with its flecks of red bell pepper, juicy pink shrimp, and brightly colored carrots, looks as good as it tastes.

Makes 4 servings

2 heads Romaine lettuce,
    torn into pieces
½ medium onion, chopped
    (about ½ cup)
1 red bell pepper, cut into strips
    (about 1 cup)

2 carrots, grated (about ½ cup)
24 cooked shrimp
Caesar Dressing (page 171)

Divide the lettuce among 4 dinner plates. Top each plate with equal portions of onion, bell pepper, carrot, and shrimp. Drizzle 1 tablespoon of dressing over each salad and serve.

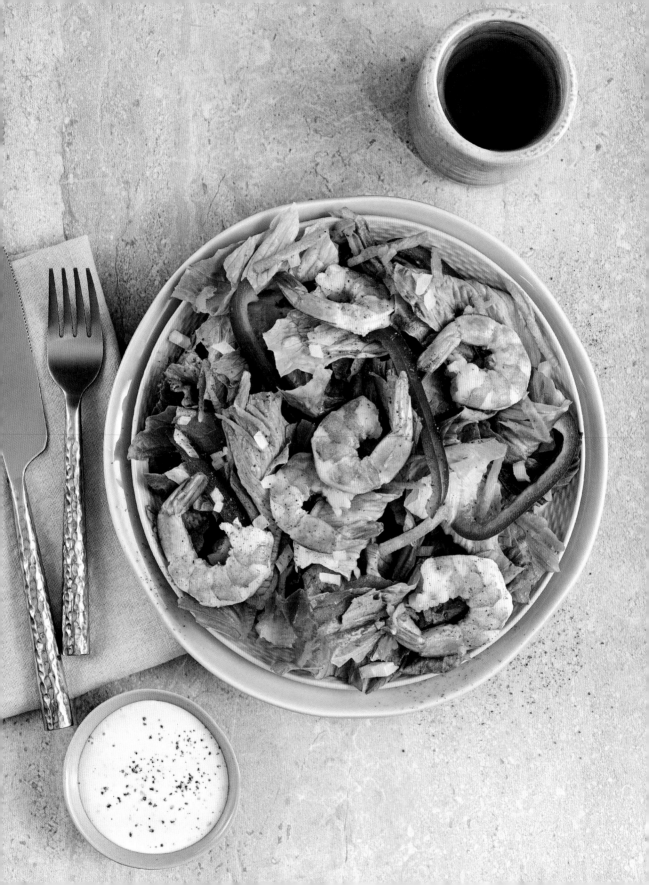

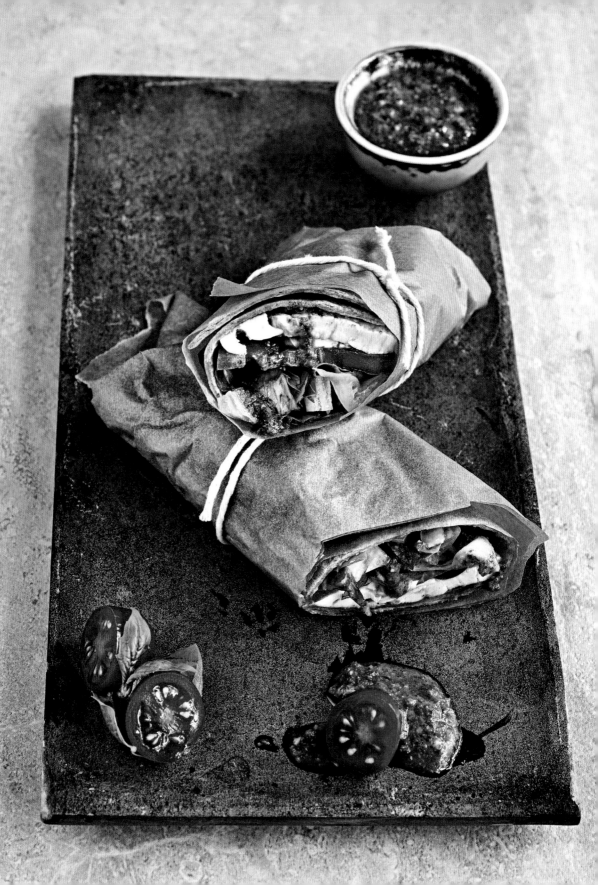

MEDITERRANEAN WRAPS WITH GARDEN PESTO

These wraps are great to pack and carry for a picnic in the park, lunch at your office, or that long drive or plane ride when you don't want to buy food at the airport or at a rest stop along the road.

Makes 4 servings

FOR THE PESTO

1 clove garlic

⅓ cup walnuts, chopped

¼ cup grated Parmesan cheese

2 cups well-packed fresh basil

½ teaspoon salt

⅓ cup extra-virgin olive oil

FOR THE WRAPS

4 low-carb flour tortillas

8 ounces fresh mozzarella cheese, sliced into 8 thin slices

2 Roma tomatoes, sliced into 8 thin slices

Several leaves of arugula or other green leafy vegetable

MAKE THE PESTO

In a blender or food processor, combine the garlic, walnuts, cheese, basil, and salt. Slowly pour in the oil as you pulse the ingredients until they combine into a paste. Add a little more oil, if necessary, to make a smooth paste. Transfer to a bowl.

MAKE THE WRAPS

Spread each tortilla with about 6 tablespoons of the pesto. Top with 2 slices of cheese, 2 slices of tomato, and a few leaves of arugula. Roll each tortilla tightly into a wrap and serve. Refrigerate any leftover pesto for up to 3 days.

SALAD DRESSINGS

ITALIAN DRESSING

Makes ½ cup

2 tablespoons white vinegar

2 tablespoons chopped fresh parsley

1 tablespoon fresh lemon juice

1 teaspoon dried basil

Pinch dried oregano

2 cloves garlic, minced

6 tablespoons extra-virgin olive oil

Salt and freshly ground pepper

In a small mixing bowl, whisk together the vinegar, parsley, lemon juice, basil, oregano, and garlic. Add the olive oil in a steady stream while whisking. Add salt and pepper to taste. Serve immediately over fresh greens.

VINAIGRETTE

Makes ½ cup

1 teaspoon Dijon mustard

1 teaspoon minced fresh garlic

2 tablespoons champagne vinegar

1 teaspoon salt

½ teaspoon black pepper

½ cup extra-virgin olive oil

In a small bowl, whisk together the mustard, garlic, vinegar, salt, and pepper. While whisking, slowly add the olive oil until the vinaigrette is emulsified.

RASPBERRY VINAIGRETTE

Makes 1 cup

½ cup white wine vinegar

¼ cup extra-virgin olive oil

¼ cup fresh raspberries

2 teaspoons honey

Combine all the ingredients in blender or food processor and blend until smooth. Store in the fridge for up to 4 days, though it is best when used freshly made.

CAESAR DRESSING

Makes 1¾ cups

2 cloves garlic, finely chopped

2 tablespoons lemon juice

2 teaspoons Dijon mustard

2 teaspoons Worcestershire sauce

1 cup mayonnaise

⅓ cup extra-virgin olive oil

½ cup shredded Parmesan cheese

1 teaspoon anchovy paste

¼ teaspoon ground black pepper

Combine the garlic, lemon juice, mustard, and Worcestershire sauce in a medium bowl. Whisk in the mayonnaise, olive oil, cheese, anchovy paste, and pepper until thoroughly combined.

Coda

I think dinner puts a nice, final flourish on the day. Cooking allows you to decompress, giving you a little break from work, studies, and all the other to-dos that fill your mind. And if you're sitting down with friends and family, dinner gives you a chance to catch up with the ones you love and get rejuvenated physically—and emotionally—for the next day.

FLOUNDER WITH SAUTÉED KALE

This was the first dish I taught Olu to make. Flounder is a light fish that cooks quickly and doesn't need a ton of seasoning to bring out its pleasant flavor. Kale is my faux version of collard greens. Collards are my favorite dish to make on holidays, but they take a while to cook. I used to drop in a ham hock or turkey leg back when I was still eating meat, but now I can satisfy my collards cravings with this kale recipe any day of the week, and I enjoy having it with the flounder instead of poultry or pork.

Makes 4 to 5 servings

FOR THE KALE

2 tablespoons extra-virgin olive oil

1 onion, diced, preferably yellow

1 tablespoon crushed red pepper, or as much as you like

4 cloves garlic, diced

2 bundles kale

4 cups low-sodium vegetable broth

Splash white wine vinegar

Salt and pepper

Hot sauce

FOR THE FLOUNDER

2 tablespoons extra-virgin olive oil

2 fillets flounder

Salt and pepper

MAKE THE KALE

Heat a large pot over high heat.

Drizzle the olive oil into the pot. Add the chopped onion and cook until it turns translucent, about 3 to 4 minutes.

Add the crushed red pepper and garlic. Cook until the garlic turns fragrant, about 1 minute.

Tear the kale leaves right off the spine with your hands so that the leaves are in equal-size pieces, and add the kale to the pot. Pour the vegetable broth over the kale and bring to a boil.

Add the white wine vinegar along with salt and pepper. Reduce the heat to a simmer and let cook for 40 minutes.

Using tongs or a slotted spoon, place the sautéed kale on a plate and add hot sauce to taste.

MAKE THE FLOUNDER

About 15 minutes before the kale is finished cooking, prepare the flounder. Heat the oil in a medium nonstick skillet over medium-high heat. Season the fish with salt and pepper and add it to the skillet, skin side up. Cook until golden brown, about 3 minutes. Turn the fish over and continue cooking 2 to 3 minutes more. Remove the fish from the skillet and serve immediately over the sautéed kale.

Opening-Night Gala

Nourishing your body, enjoying a flavorful meal, and spending time with loved ones are all special moments. So why not make dining at home as festive, fun, and elegant as eating out? Food is fuel, but eating is also a pleasure.

- Set aside the plastic jug, and fill a graceful carafe with water instead. Drink your H_2O out of a wineglass.
- Buy a set of colorful dishes. Then, instead of saving them for the holidays, recognize that every day you are alive and working toward your goals is an occasion worth celebrating. Use your "good china" to plate your Act 1 and Act 2 foods.
- Even if you're in a dorm room, eating off a tray, or at a desk that also functions as your kitchen table, make it beautiful. Decorate it with candles, or fill a cup or vase with your favorite flowers.

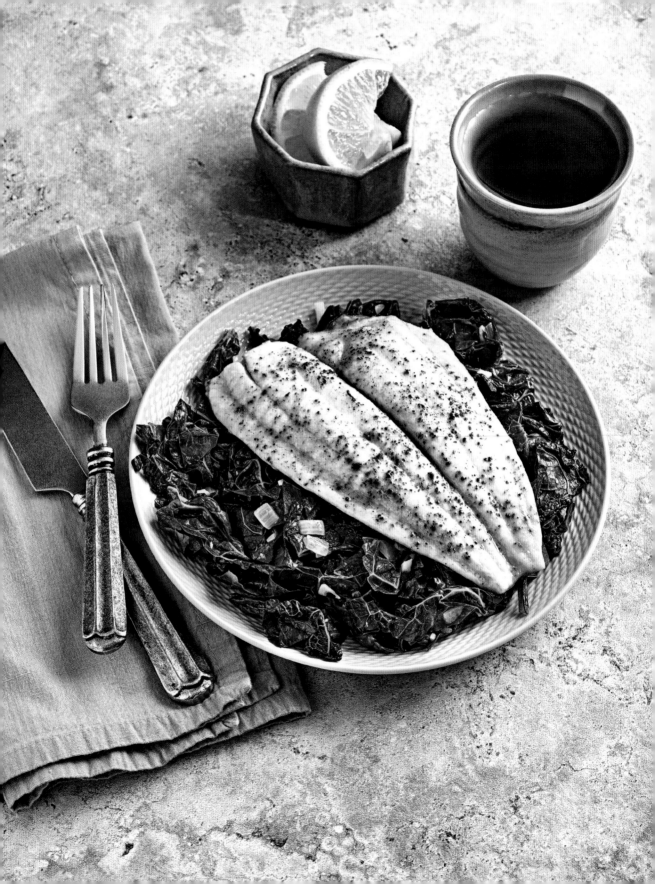

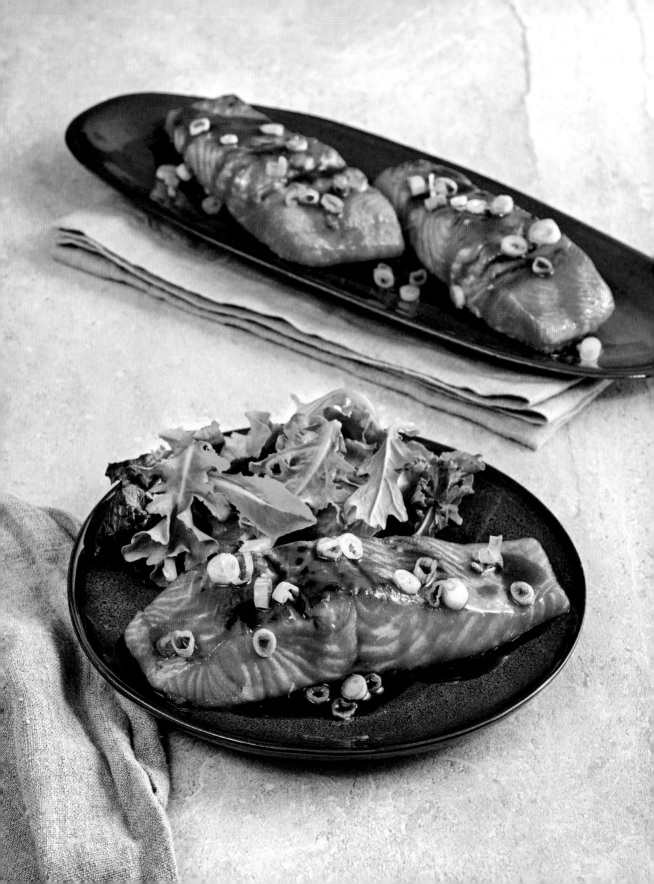

CITRUS SALMON

This light, flavorful fish dish has become a real staple in my dinner repertoire. It's Olu's favorite meal, and I've cooked it so often I could probably make it in my sleep! One of the joys of cooking is being able to improvise, and so I vary the amount of each ingredient I put in the citrus marinade. I taste and adjust the recipe to whatever I prefer that day. I also like to give the sauce, made from the marinade, a lot of time to simmer so that it has a chance to really thicken. I'll have it on the stove, bubbling away, while the fish is broiling.

Makes 4 servings

1 cup orange juice

1 cup brown sugar, packed

¾ cup low-sodium soy sauce

1 tablespoon ground white pepper

1 teaspoon salt

1 tablespoon white wine vinegar

1 bunch scallions, thinly sliced

1 pound salmon fillets, skin on

Combine the orange juice, brown sugar, soy sauce, pepper, salt, vinegar, and scallions in a large bowl and whisk well.

Pour about half of this mixture into a baking dish and add the salmon fillets, making sure they are completely covered with the marinade. Cover and refrigerate for 20 minutes.

Preheat the broiler while the salmon is marinating.

Pour the remaining marinade mixture into a small saucepan. Cook over low heat for 25 to 30 minutes, until thickened.

Cover the bottom of an oven-safe casserole dish with a tiny bit of the liquid in which the salmon was marinated. (Discard the rest of the marinade liquid.) Place the marinated salmon in the dish, skin side down, and broil for about 12 minutes, or until the salmon flakes when tested with a fork.

Pour the sauce over the salmon and serve immediately.

MASHED BUTTERNUT SQUASH

This dish may remind you of candied yams with its syrupy sweetness and creamy texture, but it packs fewer calories. It's a great side dish to flounder or another light fish. It's also filling and satisfying enough to enjoy all on its own.

Makes 4 servings

1 large butternut squash, peeled

⅓ cup maple syrup

½ teaspoon salt

¼ teaspoon pepper

2 tablespoons half-and-half

Cut the squash into 1- to 2-inch cubes and place them in a large pot. Fill the pot with enough water to cover the squash by about an inch. Bring to a boil over high heat. Cover and reduce the heat to medium-low; simmer until the squash is tender, about 10 to 25 minutes or until you can pierce it easily with a fork.

Drain the squash and transfer it to a mixing bowl. Add the syrup, salt, pepper, and half-and-half. Mash with a potato masher or electric mixer until the squash is the consistency of mashed potatoes.

QUICK SALSA CHILI

This hearty chili is great to eat on a cold evening. It includes tofu instead of meat, but you can also choose to skip the protein entirely and just savor the flavors of the veggies and spices.

Makes 4 servings

Vegetable cooking spray

1 pound ground tofu

1 medium green bell pepper, chopped (about 1 cup)

2 cups chunky salsa

1 (15-ounce) can tomato sauce

1 tablespoon chili powder

1 teaspoon cumin

1 (15-ounce) can kidney beans, rinsed and drained

Salt and pepper

Spray a skillet with cooking spray. Add the tofu and cook over medium heat until browned, about 6 to 8 minutes.

Transfer the tofu to a soup pot. Add the bell pepper, salsa, tomato sauce, chili powder, cumin, and beans, and season with salt and pepper. Cover, increase the heat to high, and bring to a boil.

Reduce the heat and simmer for 20 minutes. Ladle into 4 soup bowls and serve.

MOROCCAN SCALLOPS WITH QUINOA

This dish resembles a light stew and features some of the foods I love most. The quinoa, a great fiber-filled alternative to white rice, goes well with the delicate flavor of the scallops. The figs lend just a hint of sweetness, and the pungent spices—cardamom, turmeric, ginger—transport you to a faraway place.

Makes 4 servings

½ teaspoon turmeric

½ teaspoon ginger

¼ teaspoon ground cinnamon

¼ teaspoon cardamom

4 tablespoons extra-virgin olive oil

½ medium onion, preferably yellow, chopped (about ½ cup)

1½ pounds sea scallops, patted dry

3 cups low-sodium vegetable broth

1 cup white cooking wine

6 well-packed cups baby spinach

8 dried Mission figs, chopped

1 cup uncooked quinoa

Salt and pepper

Combine the turmeric, ginger, cinnamon, and cardamom in a small bowl.

Heat the olive oil in a large skillet over medium heat. Add the onion and sauté until tender, about 5 minutes. Add the spice blend and sauté for another 30 seconds.

Increase the heat to medium-high. Add the scallops to the skillet, and cook until tender—about 2 minutes on each side. Add 1 cup of the broth and the wine to the skillet. Reduce the heat and simmer. After about 3 minutes, stir in the spinach and figs. Cook until the spinach is wilted, about 2 minutes. Turn off the heat. Drain off and discard excess liquid.

Place the quinoa and the remaining 2 cups vegetable broth in a medium saucepan. Cover the saucepan and bring to a boil, then reduce the heat and simmer until the quinoa is tender and circles appear around the grain, usually when all of the liquid is absorbed—12 to 15 minutes. Remove from the heat.

Portion the scallop and spinach mixture and the quinoa onto 4 plates. Season each dish with salt and pepper to taste.

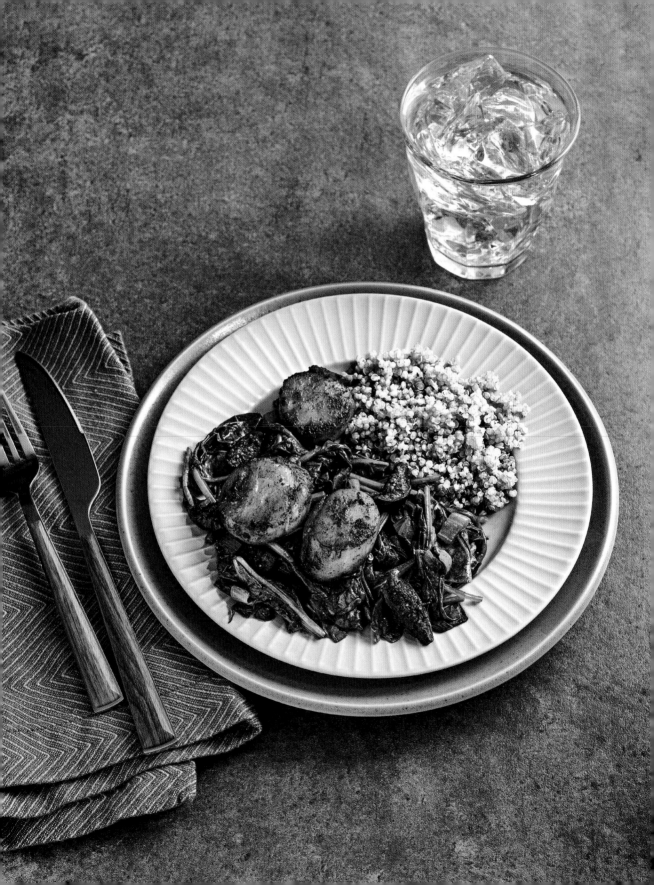

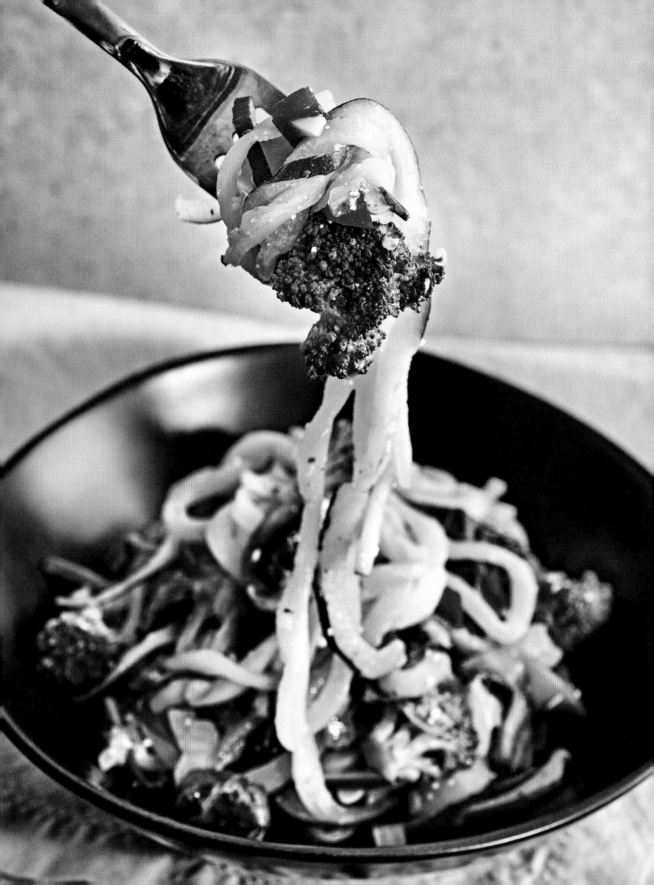

ZOODLES PRIMAVERA

This dish allows you to satisfy your pasta cravings but substitutes delicious vegetables—zucchini, spinach, and broccoli—for the pasta. With the addition of Italian seasoning, garlic, and Parmesan cheese, I don't think you'll miss the spaghetti!

Makes 4 servings

4 medium zucchinis, ends trimmed

4 tablespoons extra-virgin olive oil

2 cloves garlic, minced

1 small onion, chopped
(about ½ cup)

1 cup broccoli florets

2 cups spinach, tightly packed

½ cup sliced mushrooms

½ red bell pepper, chopped
(about ½ cup)

Salt and pepper

1 teaspoon dried Italian spices
(typically a medley of basil,
oregano, rosemary, onion
powder, and garlic powder—
available in a jar)

½ cup grated Parmesan cheese

Special equipment: Spiralizer

To create the "zoodles," insert the zucchini into the spiralizer, one at a time, much like you'd sharpen a pencil. (Please follow the manufacturer's instructions.) Set aside the vegetable noodles.

In a large skillet, heat the olive oil over medium-high heat. Add the garlic and onion and cook until translucent, about 4 to 5 minutes. Add the broccoli, spinach, mushrooms, and bell pepper. Sprinkle with salt and pepper. Cook on medium, stirring frequently, for 5 to 7 minutes, or until the vegetables are just tender.

Add the spiralized zucchini and dried Italian spices. Continue cooking for another 5 minutes, stirring frequently. Top with the cheese and serve.

TOFU-VEGGIE STIR-FRY

You can whip this stir-fry up faster than it would take to get a delivery of takeout. If you prefer seafood to tofu, you can use shrimp instead.

Makes 4 servings

1 tablespoon sesame oil

½ onion, chopped

2 teaspoons minced garlic

1 (16-ounce) package tofu, drained and cut into cubes, or 2 cups shrimp, peeled and deveined

Asian vegetables such as snow peas or bok choy chopped into 1- to 2-inch pieces

½ teaspoon crushed red pepper

½ cup low-sodium vegetable broth

3 tablespoons honey

2 tablespoons low-sodium soy sauce

1 tablespoon cornstarch dissolved in ¼ cup cold water

In a large skillet, heat the oil over medium-high heat, stir in the onion, and cook until tender. Stir in the garlic and cook for 30 seconds. Stir in the tofu. Sauté until golden brown, 1 to 2 minutes. If using shrimp, add the shrimp, cook for 2 to 3 minutes, then flip and cook for a few minutes more, until the shrimp are opaque.

Stir in the vegetables and crushed red pepper and heat through. Turn off the heat and let sit while you make the sauce.

In a small saucepan, combine the broth, honey, and soy sauce. Mix well and bring to a simmer on medium heat. Cook for 2 minutes. Stir in the cornstarch-water mixture. Continue to simmer until the sauce thickens, stirring constantly. Remove from the heat.

Divide the tofu-vegetable mixture into 4 portions and place on plates. Pour the sauce over the tofu and vegetables and serve immediately.

COCONUT QUINOA
AND LENTIL CURRY

This dish combines some of my favorite ingredients and flavors, from the brightness of the coconut oil to the earthy taste of the lentils to the heat of the curry powder. The lime, red curry paste, and soy sauce make a nice medley of savory and sour. With fresh naan on the side, you have a whole meal.

Makes 4 servings

2 tablespoons coconut oil

2 red bell peppers, chopped

2 to 3 carrots, chopped

2 cloves garlic, minced or grated

2 to 3 tablespoons Thai red curry paste (I like to use 3)

1 tablespoon curry powder (I like spicy curry powder)

1 (14-ounce) can full-fat coconut milk

4 cups coconut water or low-sodium vegetable broth or water

1 tablespoon fish sauce, or soy sauce if vegan

1 cup green lentils, rinsed

1 cup mixed red and white quinoa

3 to 4 big handfuls baby kale

Zest and juice from ½ lemon

¼ cup chopped fresh cilantro

¼ cup chopped fresh basil

1 mango, sliced or chopped

Zest and juice from 1 lime

Greek yogurt, 1 chopped Fresno chili, and ⅓ cup chopped almonds for topping

Fresh naan (available at most grocery stores)

Heat the coconut oil in a large heavy-bottomed pot set over medium heat.

Once the oil is hot, add the bell peppers and carrots, and cook for 2 to 3 minutes, or until lightly charred on the edges. Add the garlic and cook for 30 seconds.

Add the Thai red curry paste and curry powder, and continue cooking for another minute, or until the curry is fragrant. Slowly pour in the coconut milk, coconut water, and fish sauce. Stir to combine and then bring the mixture to a boil.

Once the mixture is boiling, stir in the lentils and quinoa.

Reduce the heat to a simmer, cover, and cook for 20 to 25 minutes, or until the lentils are tender and the quinoa is soft. Stir in the kale and continue cooking, uncovered, for another 5 minutes. Remove from the heat and stir in the lemon juice and zest, cilantro, and basil.

Ladle the curry into bowls and top with mango. Drizzle the mango with the lime juice and sprinkle on the zest. Garnish the curry with a dollop of Greek yogurt, the chopped Fresno chili, and almonds. Serve with the fresh naan.

Cut the Salt. Reach for the Herbs.

Rather than adding a bunch of salt to your food, cook with garlic, onions, and fresh herbs instead. They add so much flavor to your dish that your palate will appreciate all those new tastes, and after a while, you probably won't want to reach for the saltshaker. Cutting down on sodium is good for your health and reduces bloat as well. I used to eat a bag of salted and shelled sunflower seeds at night after dinner because I thought it was a light, healthy snack. I would wake up with a bloated stomach and swollen eyes. I'm especially sensitive to salt, but I think it's a good idea for most of us to cut back on sodium—especially at night. And drink plenty of water!

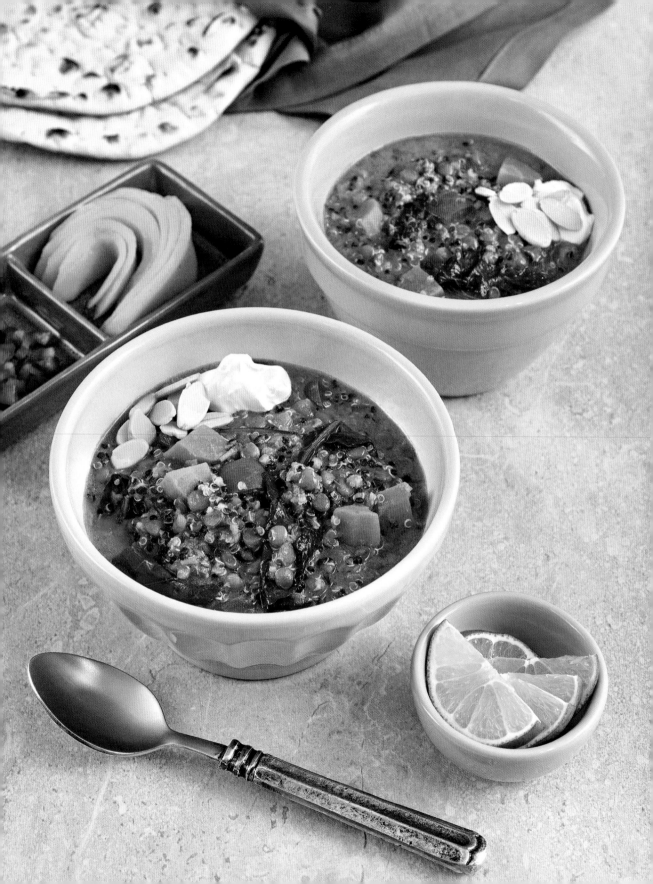

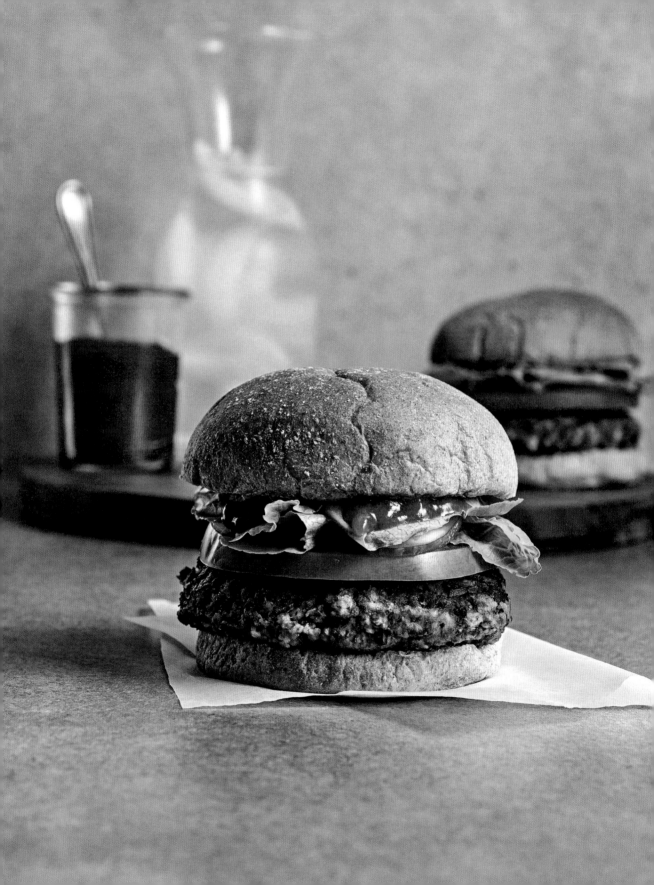

ULTIMATE VEGGIE BURGERS

These are so flavorful, with garlic, black beans, and spices, that even if you're a meat eater, I don't think you'll mind skipping the turkey or beef patty on the bun. Consider adding these burgers to your Fourth of July cookout menu to give your guests a different treat, and you can use whatever condiments you like—though you probably won't need them!

Makes 4 servings

½ medium onion, chopped
    (about ½ cup)
4 cloves garlic, minced
    (about 1 tablespoon)
2 (15-ounce) cans black beans,
    rinsed, drained, and patted dry
    with a paper towel

1 teaspoon cumin
½ teaspoon crushed red pepper
1 egg
¾ cup panko bread crumbs
Salt and pepper
Vegetable cooking spray
4 whole wheat hamburger rolls

Add the onion, garlic, half of the black beans, and the cumin, crushed red pepper, and egg to a blender or food processor and pulse to combine. Transfer the mixture to a large bowl.

In a small bowl, mash the remaining beans with a fork. Season with salt and pepper to taste. Add these beans and the bread crumbs to the onion-bean mixture. Mix until well combined.

Divide the mixture into 4 portions and form into patties. Spray a skillet with cooking spray. Place the patties on the skillet and cook them over medium-high heat for about 5 minutes on each side, or until cooked through.

Serve on hamburger buns with your favorite toppings: sliced tomato, lettuce, onion, pickles, ketchup, or mustard.

Sides, Soups, Snacks, and More

Depending on the moment and your mood, you may not want to indulge in a full meal, but you might still be craving something light to nibble on. On a cold evening, you may just want a hearty bowl of soup, or some sweet potato fries to munch on while you're watching your favorite TV show. The great thing about these light bites is that they can give you a little energy boost while also quelling your hunger, keeping you from overeating later. So there's no reason to feel guilty about snacking!

HIGH-FIBER BLENDER JAM

There's nothing like homemade jam. This one relies on the natural sugars inside the fruits. It tastes great slathered on muffins, toast, croissants, or any other breakfast bread. It can also be stirred into plain Greek yogurt as a natural sweetener.

Makes about 3 cups

1 cup chopped dried unsweetened apricots

1 cup dried cranberries

1 to 1½ cups unsweetened prune juice

1 cup chopped pitted prunes

1 cup chopped dried Mission figs

Place the apricots and cranberries in a blender, along with ½ cup of the prune juice. Blend until smooth. Add the prunes, figs, and the remaining ½ to 1 cup prune juice. Blend well, stopping the blender and stirring occasionally to ensure that all the ingredients are blended. Add more prune juice, if necessary, to ensure that the final consistency is that of a jam (it should cling to a spoon and not be runny).

Transfer the jam to a container with a top. Keep in the refrigerator. The jam should last about 1 month.

MISTY'S RAW BARRES

These "barres" have everything—coconut, fruit, nuts, and chocolate. What's not to love?

Makes 8 to 10 bars

1 cup Medjool dates, pitted, chopped, and soaked in water to soften them

1 cup raw cashews

½ cup hemp seeds

½ cup sesame seeds

¼ cup raw cacao powder

Pinch sea salt

2 tablespoons coconut oil, melted

¼ cup almond butter

1 tablespoon vanilla extract

½ cup unsweetened coconut flakes

½ cup dried cherries

Remove dates from soaking water and pat dry. Combine the dates, cashews, seeds, cacao powder, and sea salt in a food processor (or a strong blender). Pulse and process all the ingredients together until the texture is coarse.

Add the coconut oil, almond butter, and vanilla. Pulse again until the mixture reaches a dough-like consistency. Remove from the blender or processor and place in a medium mixing bowl. Stir in the coconut and cherries. Mix well.

Transfer the mixture to an 8-by-12-inch baking dish. Place in the freezer for 30 minutes to harden. Cut into bars, and store in an airtight container in the refrigerator for up to 1 week.

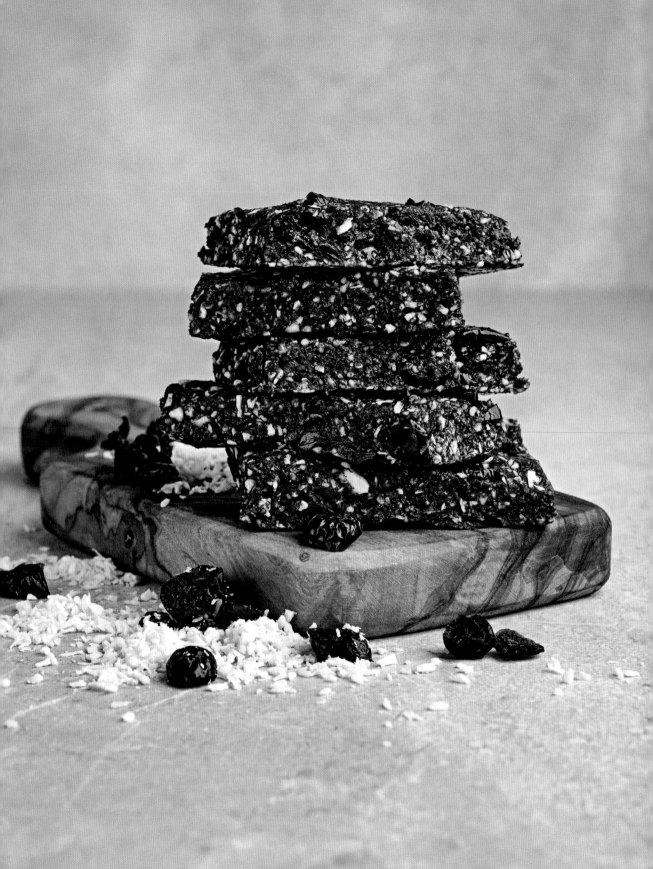

LOADED MOCK POTATO SOUP

Cauliflower is a great potato substitute, offering a similar texture but fewer calories. You can chop it up and mix it with yogurt for a lower-calorie take on mashed potatoes, or toss it with onion and garlic to make this wonderful soup.

Makes 4 to 6 servings

1 medium cauliflower, cut into small chunks
1 medium onion, diced
1 clove garlic, minced
6 cups low-sodium vegetable broth

½ cup Greek yogurt
2 tablespoons extra-virgin olive oil
Salt and pepper
¾ cup shredded Swiss cheese
4 tablespoons chopped fresh chives

Place the cauliflower, onion, garlic, and broth in a large soup pot on high heat. Bring to a boil.

Reduce the heat to low. Cover and simmer until the cauliflower is very tender, about 20 minutes.

Puree the mixture in a blender with the yogurt (in batches, if necessary), being careful with the hot liquid, until completely smooth and thick. Transfer the mixture back to the soup pot, and heat over medium-low. Add the olive oil and mix well. Add salt and pepper to taste. Stir in the cheese and let it melt.

Ladle the soup into 4 large bowls, and garnish with the chives.

Note: This soup also makes a great base for clams. Add 2 to 3 cans of clams (drained) to the soup prior to serving, heat the soup, and you have a light clam chowder.

SWEET POTATO FRIES

Sweet potatoes are a great side for so many dishes. Instead of eating more traditional French fries, which are doused in oil, try this sweet potato version, which goes in the oven and is spritzed with a little cooking spray. I like to sprinkle these fries with salt and paprika, or sometimes I use paprika and my version of House Seasoning.

Makes 4 servings and 1½ cups House Seasoning

FOR THE FRIES

2 large sweet potatoes, peeled

Vegetable cooking spray

½ teaspoon salt (optional, instead of House Seasoning)

½ teaspoon paprika (optional, instead of House Seasoning)

Reduced-sugar ketchup or agave nectar ketchup (optional)

FOR THE HOUSE SEASONING

2 teaspoons salt

½ teaspoon black pepper

½ teaspoon garlic powder

MAKE THE FRIES

Preheat the oven to 450°F.

Cut the sweet potatoes in half lengthwise; then cut each half into 4 long spears.

Spray a baking sheet with cooking spray, and place spears in a single layer.

Spray the spears with cooking spray. Bake for 15 to 20 minutes; then flip the spears over with a spatula. Bake for another 10 minutes, or until the potatoes are lightly browned.

MAKE THE HOUSE SEASONING

Mix together the salt, pepper, and garlic.

Remove the sweet potatoes from the oven, and sprinkle them lightly with salt and paprika or with 1 tablespoon House Seasoning. Serve immediately with ketchup if desired.

Store the leftover House Seasoning in an airtight jar in your pantry or spice rack.

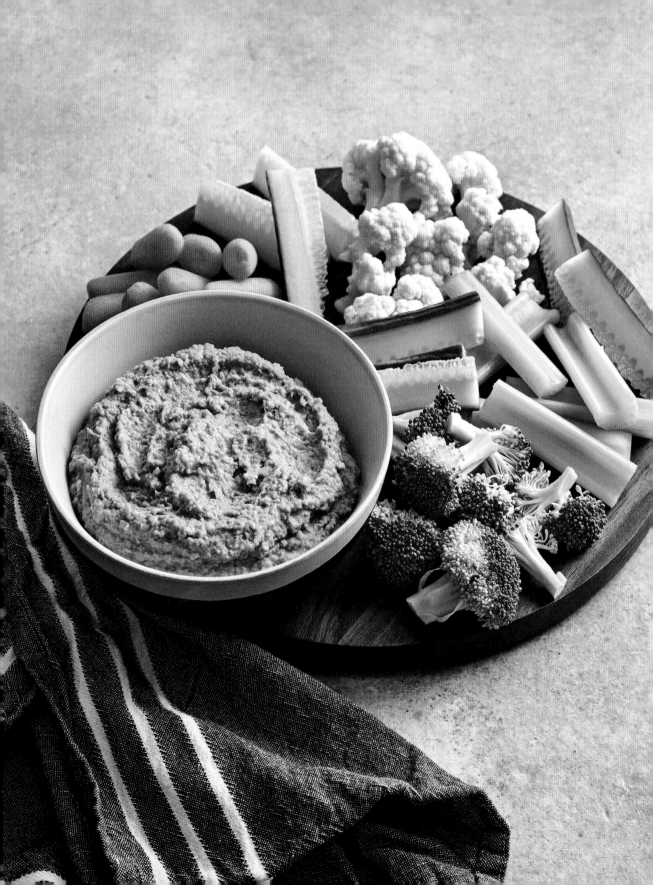

YUMMUS AND VEGGIES

This is my take on hummus. Instead of garbanzo beans, I use green peas and toss in a little red bell pepper. It makes for a colorful dip but still has that traditional hummus flavor thanks to the tahini.

Makes 4 servings (½ cup each)

2 cups fresh peas, cooked

1 small onion, diced

1 clove garlic, minced

1 tablespoon tahini
(sesame seed butter)

½ teaspoon salt

¼ cup extra-virgin olive oil, plus
more if needed for consistency

½ red bell pepper, diced

Place the peas, onion, garlic, tahini, salt, and ¼ cup of olive oil in a blender or food processor. Puree until the mixture becomes a thick paste. If the mixture is too thick, add more olive oil, 1 teaspoon at a time, until it reaches the right consistency.

Transfer to 4 small bowls. Sprinkle each serving with the diced bell pepper.

Use the Yummus for dipping with fresh cut raw vegetables: baby carrots, broccoli, cauliflower, cucumber, celery, and so on.

KALE CHIPS

I'm a kale lover. I'll eat it in any form I can get. Chips were actually the first way I ever prepared it.

It's a simple, quick, tasty snack. My close friend, Jennifer, isn't a big vegetable eater, but she loves these chips. I also think it's a great recipe for kids!

Makes 2 to 4 servings

2 bundles fresh kale, washed, de-stemmed, and chopped into 1- or 2-inch pieces

2 to 3 tablespoons extra-virgin olive oil

2 to 3 tablespoons apple cider vinegar

Sea salt

Place an oven rack on the lowest shelf, and preheat the oven to 350°F.

Place the kale in a large bowl. Drizzle it lightly with the olive oil and vinegar. Toss to coat the kale completely.

Spread the kale on one large baking sheet. Bake for 10 minutes.

Remove the kale from the oven, and stir to give every piece of kale a chance to crisp.

Bake for another 10 minutes, until the kale is crispy to the touch and slightly browned. Sprinkle with sea salt and serve immediately.

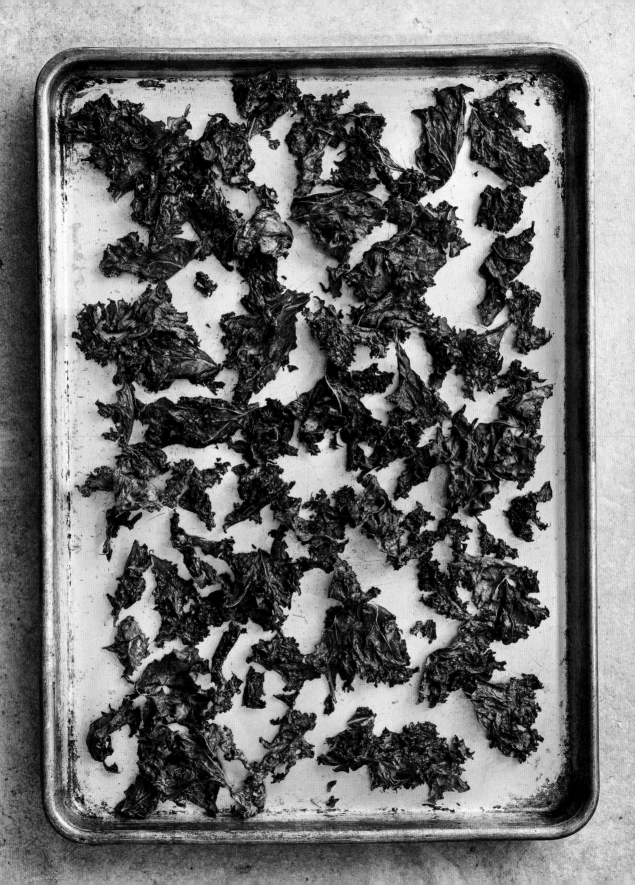

Desserts

I've made it pretty clear that I've got a serious sweet tooth, and even though I can't go overboard, devouring boxes of doughnuts like I did years ago, I still indulge from time to time. There are ways to make your treats healthier but still tasty, using fruit or agave syrup for sweetness, or perhaps almond meal instead of white flour. You're not going to sacrifice a single ounce of deliciousness.

MISTY AND MAKEDA'S BANANA OATMEAL COOKIES

My mentee Makeda and I love to share healthy recipes. She shared this one with me and we've made it together. You can use either old or fresh bananas. And feel free to improvise, adding enough oatmeal to thicken your "batter" and one or two tasty extras like pieces of a white or dark chocolate bar.

Makes 6 to 8 cookies

Vegetable cooking spray

1 cup oats, instant or regular, chopped fine

2 large ripe bananas

Preheat the oven to 350°F. Spray a baking sheet with cooking spray.

Mix the oats and bananas together, mashing the fruit with a fork. Toss in whatever extras you like. I'd suggest ¾ cup of white or dark chocolate pieces or chips.

Spoon the mixture by heaping tablespoons onto the prepared baking sheet. Bake for 15 minutes. Remove the pan from the oven, flip the cookies over, and put back in the oven to bake for another 10 minutes or until golden brown.

FRUIT AND NUT MEDLEY

I love dried fruit and nuts. They satisfy my sweets cravings and give me an energy jolt when I'm on a break from rehearsal. Having this mixture already prepared makes it easy for you to grab a quick, healthy snack instead of reaching for a bowl of ice cream or cookies.

Makes 4 servings (2 cups)

½ cup raw almonds

½ cup walnuts

½ cup raisins

¼ cup chopped dates

¼ cup coconut flakes, unsweetened

Combine all the ingredients in a mixing bowl. Store in an airtight container for up to 2 weeks.

JUICES AND SMOOTHIES

CARROT JUICE

This juice is so refreshing, and it has a natural sweetness that can satisfy your sweet tooth. I mix it up with a little apple and lemon, which gives it an added brightness. It's perfect on a warm summer afternoon, or I'll fix a big glass and sip it on the couch when I get home from class and rehearsals at ABT.

Makes 2 servings

1 pound carrots, cut into chunks
1 large apple, cut into chunks

1 small lemon, peeled and deseeded

Toss the carrots, apple, and lemon into a blender or juicer. Blend or juice until smooth—about 5 to 6 minutes.

BALLERINA SMOOTHIE

This is a power booster in a blender! The spinach and berries give you a potpourri of vitamins. Add the almond or coconut milk, and it becomes a super-healthy milk shake.

Makes 1 serving

½ cup berries (any type)
1 handful baby spinach
1 cup nondairy milk (such as almond milk or coconut milk)

2 teaspoons honey or agave syrup (optional)

Place all the ingredients in a blender and blend until smooth. Serve in a tall glass and enjoy.

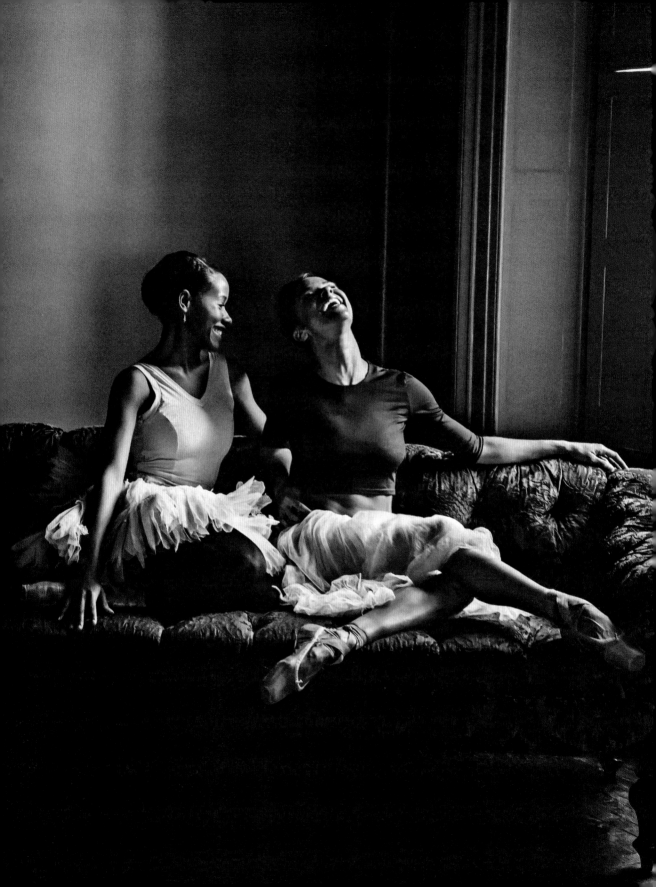

PART 4

Mentors

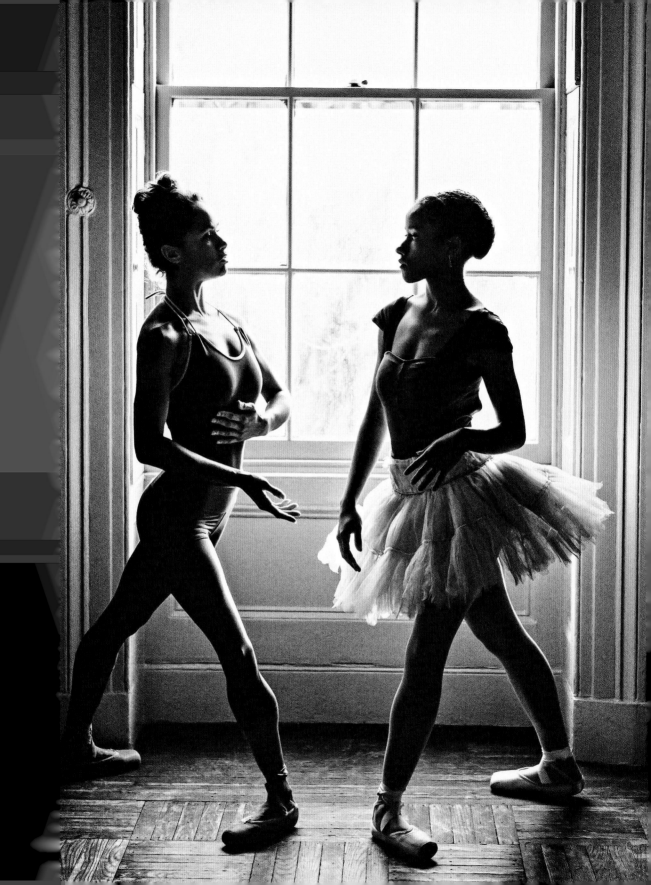

Chapter 11

MASTER CLASS

Having mentors and role models in our lives is essential. They can light our way, providing guidance, support, and inspiration to help us achieve whatever goal we are striving for, be it better fitness, more robust health, a different career path, or simply—crucially—a more centered and contented life.

You might emulate figures that you may never meet: inspirational speakers, writers, artists, or businesspeople. But finding someone with whom you can forge a personal connection is particularly nurturing, providing the intimacy that allows you to gain knowledge firsthand, to ask questions as you navigate the twists and turns of your own course, and to unspool your goals, fears, and dreams.

A mentor can mean the difference between giving up on a goal and pushing yourself to do things you didn't know you could and becoming someone you didn't realize you had the capability to be. Seeing your dreams and goals projected through someone else's eyes can give you immense strength.

I discovered the power of mentorship at a young age, when I would head to the Boys & Girls Club each day after school. I was surrounded by counselors who guided me through my homework lessons while my mother was working late to provide for my five siblings and me. The Boys & Girls Club was also where I was introduced to ballet and met my first ballet teacher, Cynthia Bradley.

That initial ballet class launched me on a journey that would change my life, paving the way to my future. And Cynthia assumed a role that went well beyond teaching me to dance. She became a mentor, a guide, who taught me skills that I hadn't yet developed, like how to express my opinions about the world around me. She would literally force me to speak—to sit and think about my feelings and then give voice to those thoughts and emotions. No one had ever empowered me in that way, and I began to understand then that whatever stage of life we are in, we all benefit from

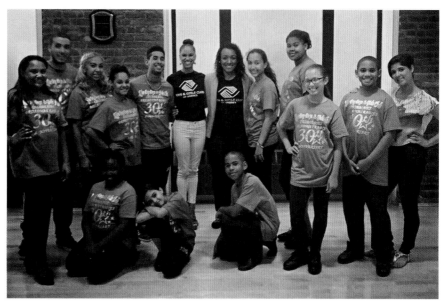
Working with Boys & Girls Club youth.

having someone in our sphere who gives us encouragement and a different perspective. Cynthia helped me to grow and set me on the path that led to my ultimate goal of dancing with American Ballet Theatre.

Later, once I had become a professional dancer, I hit a ceiling and felt that I was no longer progressing. Deep down I knew that I had the potential, but I lacked the support and confidence I needed to propel myself beyond the corps de ballet. I also struggled with the isolation I felt being a black woman in the world of classical dance.

There were two women in particular, powerful and accomplished, who guided me through this difficult time—Susan Fales-Hill and Raven Wilkinson.

Susan, a writer, producer, ABT board member, and ballet lover, helped me to understand that it was critical at this juncture in my life to surround myself with successful women who looked like me and who had reached milestones of their own amid sometimes challenging circumstances.

Then there was Raven. Here's a journal entry I wrote around the time I first learned about her.

> *More than half the battle is breaking thru the glass ceiling. Nobody knows about being the first . . . except the first.*

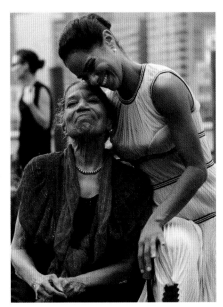
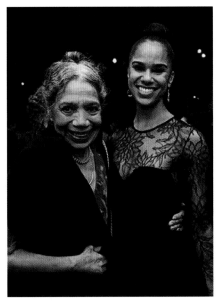

With my mentor, Raven Wilkinson.

When I joined ABT at 19 years old I knew I was passionate about ballet and that I was also different. I was a mixed-race woman with just over 5 years of ballet training under my belt. I never could have anticipated my journey and what I would later feel my purpose was. After about 6 years in the company, the article was written. The New York Times' *"Where Are All the Black Swans?" It hit me harder than I ever imagined. I learned of ballerinas I'd never heard of. Why didn't I know who they were? Why aren't they a recognized part of ballet history?*

Will I ever have a future outside of the corps de ballet? I was fortunate enough to have [actress] Victoria Rowell, Susan Fales-Hill, and [dancer] Virginia Johnson come into my life—black women who began a pattern in my life and career that would help to define my identity beyond Misty the ballerina. They gave me mentorship and encouraged me to carry on the stories of those who came before me.

At 24 years old I was promoted to the rank of soloist and I was yet to see a black woman stand next to me in the company of 80 dancers. I had no real knowledge of my place in history or in the ballet world. Stories were frequently written in the press that I was the first African American woman in ABT's history to obtain this position. I remember the day Julie Kent, principal dancer with the company, informed me that there had been another who had come before me. I was pleasantly surprised and curious. But at the time, I could find nothing while Googling black soloists with ABT. However, I would come to learn more about the contributions of African American ballerinas like Anne Benna Sims and Nora Kimball, who was the first black woman soloist at ABT.

It was soon after that the Ballet Russe de Monte Carlo documentary came out. I watched and learned of Raven Wilkinson who had danced with the company in the 1950s and was chased out of the company by the KKK. I felt an emotional attachment and connection that I didn't know I yearned for. I felt for the first time what my purpose might be in this rarified elite white world.

Raven was the first African American woman to dance with the Ballet Russe de Monte Carlo. She was a beacon of hope for me before I ever met her. Her tenacity and perseverance are greater than she'd ever let on, and she has served as an example, and an inspiration, to me as I pursue my own dreams.

———————

Whether they're providing you guidance at work or imparting nuggets of wisdom about relationships or your personal passions, mentors can emerge in any number of ways. Perhaps you meet someone whose strength or talent you respect, and you organically form a relationship. Other times, you may need to be proactive, coming straight out and asking someone whose success you admire to take you under her or his wing, to help you out, or to be a sounding board.

Either way, such relationships need to be nurtured and cultivated. Call or text when you need advice or want to learn details about your mentor's personal trek. And don't underestimate the importance of face time. Nothing beats the power of being able to share laughter and conversation in person, so be sure to ask your mentor out to lunch or out for coffee, or to meet after school on occasion.

Many professionals believe that mentors are critical in the workplace to help you understand all the corporate rules and codes in order to ensure that your many talents get the chance to shine, and to help you sidestep potential minefields. But there is value in having a mentor long before you apply for a job, begin your climb up the corporate ladder, or launch a business.

Maybe as a high school freshman, you observe an older student who's running for student government or starting a group on campus. Think about asking her to grab a mocha latte (with soy milk!) or approaching her in the cafeteria to ask for her tips on leadership or on how she stays organized. Or perhaps one of your peers is excelling in a class where you struggle. Ask if she or he would be willing to study with you sometime.

As you're pursuing your college studies, you'll no doubt have an interest in various career paths. And why not? It's a ripe time to explore. Seek out your instructors during their office hours, and if they are still working in a given field, consider asking if you can shadow them for a day. Pepper them with questions about all you want to know, and build a rapport. Those same instructors can be a conduit to internships, a reference for future opportunities, and a great source of knowledge as you make your way in the world. Similarly, a supervisor at an after-school job or internship might become a lifelong friend, cheerleader, or champion.

Mentors are worth having beyond when you are starting out in your academic or professional endeavors. Remain open at any age, at any stage, to seeking out those living the life you want to live or engaging in a passion you want to pursue. Maybe you've always wanted to share your vast love for a particular hobby, but you are terrified of addressing an audience. If you attend a local event helmed by a rousing public speaker, approach the speaker afterward. Perhaps you can exchange email addresses or phone numbers, keep in touch, and gain tips on how to overcome that trepidation.

Maybe you've been wanting to get off the corporate treadmill but can't summon the energy to complete that half-finished novel tucked in your bedside drawer. Or now that you're done writing, you don't have a clue how to go about getting your manuscript published. If an author you admire is going to appear at a local book signing, go, and don't be shy! Grab a moment during the meet and greet, or when you get up close in the signing queue, to ask them for guidance. They might be willing to take a look at your writing or even to help shepherd your project once you are finished. Who knows? It could be the beginning of a beautiful friendship.

PASSING IT ON

When you have a mentor, someone who gives you the encouragement and guidance to push your own life forward, you also have an example to follow as you enable others to pursue their passions. You can be motivated to keep striving, not just for yourself, or to make your mentor proud, but because your achievements can inspire others who may be looking up to you, whether they're your children, your students, your friends, or your colleagues. The guidance you give and the relationships you nurture ultimately create a community.

In my career, I have met so many incredible young men and women, working hard to become the finest dancers and human beings that they can be, and I've formed relationships with several of them.

The first dancer I ever mentored was a young lady I met when I was performing as a guest artist with a small ballet school in Harlem. We were staging a production of *The Nutcracker*. I performed the role of the Sugar Plum Fairy, and my mentee-to-be danced as Clara.

She was an African American girl with tremendous potential, playing a role that I had performed early in my own career. With so many parallels, I felt drawn to her and asked the young lady's teacher if I could speak with her mother.

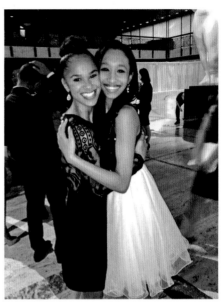

With my mentee Erica Lall, who's now in ABT's Corps de Ballet.

We had even more in common than I initially realized. I learned that she was one of ten children, and while her family was very supportive of her dancing, they were not familiar with ballet as a professional career and weren't clear how to nurture her continued study. I wanted to help.

I took her to an open audition for ABT's school, and the director loved her. I then wrote numerous emails to ABT's education department to see what the company could offer in financial help. She ended up getting a full scholarship and trained for two years with the school. We are in touch to this day.

At that same ABT school audition, a young girl shyly approached me and said I had been her role model. She and her mother asked if we could exchange contact information, and that young girl has been a mentee of mine ever since.

The number of dancers I mentor has grown steadily over the last several years, the relationships varying depending on each of their needs. Often, we are in touch via email, a way for them to ask me whatever they want and to get a speedy response no matter where in the world each of us is. They want to know so many things—how to deal with self-doubt, how to reach the next level in their dancing, what companies I think they should audition for, how to take care of themselves when they are injured, what they should eat, and, often, how to handle being a person of color in the largely white world of ballet.

Those are many of the same questions that I have asked myself, as well as my own mentors, so it makes me especially glad to be able to share some of the comfort and

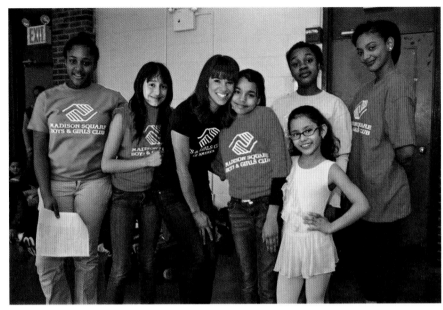

With friends at Boys & Girls Club.

guidance that have been so generously offered to me. And in passing along advice to my mentees, I am reminded during my occasional moments of doubt of all that I have learned and all that I know.

My many experiences, as a mentor, as a late-blooming dancer, as an African American ballerina, have also been instrumental to the creation of an initiative close to my heart called Project Plié.

It has been painfully clear to me how big a gap looms in the ballet world. There is a tremendous lack of diversity, and opportunities for dancers of color remain scarce. During my fifteen years as a professional ballerina, I've often wondered if the same structure that my first teacher, Cynthia, created at the Boys & Girls Club in San Pedro, could be replicated to find other young people like me, who might not have the means, access, or support to succeed in the ballet world.

ABT's former CEO Rachel Moore had a similar vision. She arrived at ABT with the idea of setting up an educational program in underprivileged communities that could nurture a new generation of dancers of color. She approached me, wanting to hear what I had experienced as a black woman throughout my training and professional career. Together, with the assistance of my manager, Gilda Squire, we came up with the idea for Project Plié. We based it on my own path, partnering with Boys & Girls Clubs all over the United States, and we are working with other ballet schools and professional companies as well.

Building Your Network

FINDING A MENTOR

- Go to your professor's office during office hours. Ask lots of questions and let her or him know your artistic or professional interests.
- Approach or send an email to a person in your chosen field whom you admire, asking if you can reach out for advice from time to time.
- Texting and Skype are great, but take your mentor out for coffee or lunch on occasion.
- Be mindful of your mentors' time. To be able to call on your mentors when you most need them, try not to overwhelm them. Maybe send an email once a month, asking how they are and giving a very brief update on how you're progressing personally or in your career. If you're in the same city, try to get together in person a couple of times a year. That way you maintain an open line of communication but don't strain the relationship or be seen as a burden.

CASTING A LIGHT: BECOMING A MENTOR

- If you're a senior in high school or college, consider being a campus guide or taking a freshman or transfer student under your wing.
- Become a part of Big Brothers Big Sisters of America.
- Be open to helping guide a student or a young person in your church, synagogue, or community who seeks you out or appears in need of support.

I've gained as much from my relationships with up-and-coming dancers as they have gained from me. Spending time with them, watching them grow in confidence and excel at their art, has been immeasurably rewarding and has given me the faith to believe that the tradition of black women in ballet, from Raven Wilkinson to Aesha Ash to Lauren Anderson to Michaela DePrince, will continue and grow ever stronger.

An entry in my journal sums up how much I feel I've been given, and how that has enabled me to share with others:

The respect, admiration, and passion I have for what I do is immense. I can't imagine having had my life take any other turn except to be a part of the ballet world. What I've gained as a student, ballerina, woman, and human being from this art form is a great understanding of how to communicate, love, grow, have compassion, and offer empathy.

Along with wanting to push myself to the highest standards I've set, I try my best to represent not only American Ballet Theatre in the best way but all of the dance world as well. Acceptance and respect from the ballet world is everything to me. Not only as a ballerina, but as an African American ballerina!

The incredible opportunities I've been given are here and exist because of ballet. For that I will forever be grateful and indebted to it. And I will forever bring the ballet world with me wherever I go, through every facet of my life. For this and for so many other reasons, I feel privileged to be a part of this community and honored to call myself a dancer!

You can create your own Project Plié. You can nurture someone else's budding talent or encourage another to live her or his best life. We all have so much to teach, and each of us has a singular perspective that can benefit those around us much more than we realize.

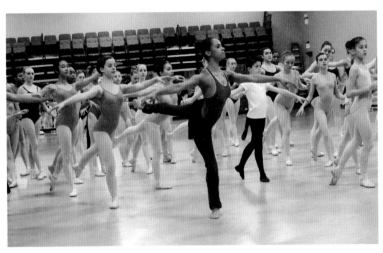

Teaching a master class.

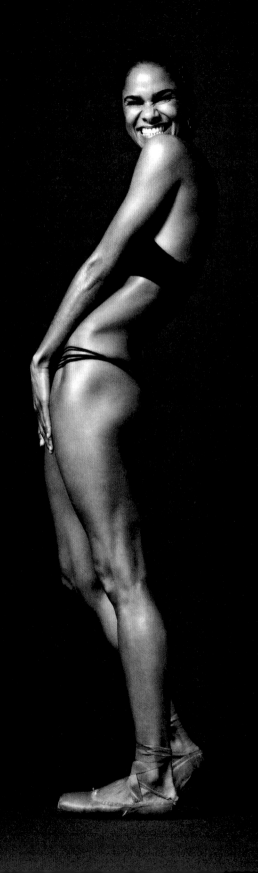

EPILOGUE

By now, you have taken steps—leaps, really—to your ideal body. You're learning to love your physique. You're eating foods that are nutritious and helping to transform your shape. You are practicing a form of exercise that helps you to channel your energy and build your mental and physical power. And your regimen of new moves is sculpting the curves and muscles that you desire.

I hope this new journey has been fun and rewarding and that you've begun to see the results that you've envisioned. But there may still be moments, days, maybe even weeks, when your motivation starts to slip. I have those times too, when I wake up in the morning and just want to stay in bed, when I'd rather go to a movie than to rehearsal, or when I can't resist having a second, third—or fourth—peanut butter cookie!

The best advice I can give is—don't give up. Getting what we desire in life takes time and effort. There are stumbles and restarts, setbacks and frustrations. And also victories.

I know when I say to keep pushing no matter what, that's easier said than done. Early in my career, not long after I became a part of ABT's corps de ballet, I suffered a stress fracture in my lower lumbar that required me to wear a brace and go through rehabilitation for an entire year. I made it back to the stage and eventually became a soloist, but it would be another eight years before I got promoted to principal. During that time, I dealt with harsh critiques of some of my performances, another debilitating injury, and, perhaps inevitably, periods of deep self-doubt that I would ever achieve my ultimate goal.

I had to take it a day, an hour, a relevé, at a time. I jotted my frustrations and fears in the pages of my journals. When I was hurt and unable to dance, I practiced my moves while lying on the floor, and I pirouetted inside my head. When criticism of my technique—sometimes fair, sometimes mean-spirited—got me down, I would think about what my giving up would mean to other young people who had been told what they couldn't do because of their skin color or background, and that would help me to rally.

I also tried to not be so hard on myself. An occasional glass of champagne or cheddar biscuit was just fine. I would carve out time to relax with friends, and I'd remind myself of all I'd learned by sharing all that I knew with my mentees, who were trying to make their own way in the dance world. I also tried to remember to pat myself on the back for triumphs large and small—when I successfully executed a series of complicated moves, when I performed a difficult role, or when I simply made more progress with a particular task than I had the day or week before.

In my journal I wrote a reflection about how great it was simply to be a part of a company that I had once dreamed about.

> *I am part of ABT! The history that will live on forever. When I'm gone that will be what lasts. Not the critics. Not the blogs. So why let that define me, distract me, scare me, make me question my purposes and ability? This is insanely rare and special. I will forever be adding layers and layers and colors to every role I've done and will do. No one started as the best or their best. All we can do is keep striving. My generation is defining ballet in America today and that is exciting.*

When you skip a day of exercise, that's not a reason to berate yourself—or a reason to abandon your workout plan altogether. Remember that tomorrow can be a new beginning, a chance to recommit to your aspirations. When you become frustrated, tap into whatever ritual gives you peace. Clear your mind, focus your energy, and once you're revived, pick up and start again.

Praise yourself for every success. When you put away the pizza menu and prepare a healthy dinner for yourself and your family instead; when you are able to run up the steps for the first time without losing your breath; when you can power through exercises that you once found difficult; when you can slip on a dress that was uncomfortable to wear. *All* of that—each and every triumph—is worth celebrating.

Our journey is as important as the finish line we are aiming for. We're on a path that is making us stronger, more centered, more focused, each and every step of the way.

Remember, it's not about fitting into a mold carved by someone else, or hitting a certain number on a bathroom scale. We all hold the power, strength, and focus to become the person we want to be, to create the body we want to have, and to carve the path we want to take. It's about being your best self—empowered, focused, healthy, and joyfully *you*!

ACKNOWLEDGMENTS

I would like to thank Charisse Jones for yet another incredibly special book. Thank you for being my voice. My gratitude to Karen Murgolo, Morgan Hedden, and Kallie Shimek for your editing efforts and patience with my wonky schedule! Thank you to Linda Duggins, who has not only attended many of my performances over the years but is now a part of my Grand Central team. Thank you to Steven Troha for continuing to be an angel in my life. Your creativity and openness is endless and inspiring. Margaret Robinson, calling on your expertise was the first step we took in creating this book. Thank you for everything. Marjorie Liebert, I don't know where I would be in my career without your words of encouragement, or where my body would be without your knowledge, which has changed my dancing. You are helping to educate a whole new audience! Gilda Squire, what can I say? The dream team. Ha ha! You are everything to me. Thank you for helping to create an opportunity that has allowed me to share my feelings about beauty, strength, quality, and intelligence in the most heartfelt way. Henry Leutwyler, you are *my* photographer. Thank you for shooting me with a style that is both real and raw. You show me as a healthy woman, ballerina, and athlete! Shubhani Sarkar, thank you for your beautiful vision for the book, and for piecing it all together so seamlessly. Amy Roth and Darcie Hunter from Gourmet Creative, your images reflect the forward thinking and boundary pushing I stand for. Thank you all.

INDEX

gratitude, 19
greens, leafy
    Mediterranean Wraps with
        Garden Pesto, 169
    Tuna Niçoise Salad, 165

H

hamstrings
    Plié en Dehors with
        Extension, 60
    Posting, 37–38, 45–46
Head, Neck, and Shoulder Roll
    exercise, 40
    variation, 44–45
herbal teas, 121
herbs, 121, 186
Hip Opener exercise, 48–49
hips
    Grand Battement, 68–72
    Hip Opener, 48–49
    Rond de Jambe, 66–67
    Walk, 60–61
honey: Bran Muffins, 152
hydration, 122

I

ideal ballerina, 96
inner thighs (adductors)
    Plié en Dehors with
        Extension, 60
    Posting, 45–46
inspiration, 11–20
intuitive power, 25–26
Italian Dressing, 170

J

Johnson, Virginia, 209
joints
    bending legs and, 77
    Grand Battement, 68–72
    Hip Opener, 48–49
    Plié, 53–57
    Rond de Jambe, 66–67
journal, 16, 18–19
    excerpts by Misty, 18, 208–10,
        215, 218
    words of appreciation for your
        body, 8
Jump exercise, 89

K

kale
    Coconut Quinoa and Lentil
        Curry, 185–86
    Flounder with Sautéed Kale,
        173–74
    Kale Chips, 198
Kent, Julie, 210
Kimball, Nora, 210
Kniaseff barre-à-terre, 15

L

Lall, Eric, 212
leeks: Lentils, 163
legs
    Adagio, 87
    Battement Dégagé, 86–87
    Battement Tendu, 83–85
    Demi-Plié, 79–81
    Grand Plié in Second
        Position, 82
    Jump, 89
    Relevé, 88
    Rond de Jambe, 66–67
Lentils, 163
Liebert, Marjorie, 15, 46, 51
Lime Shrimp, Black Bean Soup with,
    155–56
Lloyd, Carli, 14
Loaded Mock Potato Soup, 194
lunch, 126, 154
    recipes, 155–71
    Week 1, 127–30
    Week 2, 134–36
    Week 3, 139–42

M

mango: Coconut Quinoa and Lentil
    Curry, 185–86
Mashed Butternut Squash, 178
meal choreography
    breakfast, 125–26
    dinner, 126
    grocery list for three weeks,
        131
    lunch, 126
    snacks, 126
    21-Day Ballerina Body Meal
        Plan, 127–43

meals, 92–206
    Ballerina Body recipes,
        145–203
    disconnecting and, 162
    eating for energy, 105–23
    eating guidelines, 122
    eating mindfully, 162
    eating slowly, 162
    fat, dietary, 95–103
    meal choreography, 125–43
    Misty's perfect day, 123
meats, 108
meditation, 25, 28
Mediterranean Wraps with Garden
    Pesto, 169
mentors, xi, xii, 207–15
    becoming a mentor, 214
    finding a mentor, 214
    passing it on, 211–15
    Project Plié, 213, 215
mind
    affirmations, 19
    balance, 23–29
    dealing with negative thoughts
        and self-doubt, 8, 9, 13,
        18, 217–18
    embracing your body as
        perfect, 6–9
    goal-setting, 11–12, 20
    gratitude, 19
    inspiration, 11–20
    journal-keeping, 16, 18–19
    joyful movement, 26–27
    meditation, 25, 28
    motivation, 13–14
    seeking sanctuary, 29
    sticky note reminders, 8
    vision board, 17
    visualization, 14–16
    words of appreciation for your
        body, 8
mindfulness, 20, 27, 162
Misty and Makeda's Banana Oatmeal
    Cookies, 201
Moore, Rachel, 213
Moroccan Scallops with Quinoa,
    180
motivation, 13–14
    Picture, Envision, Imagine, 14
movement, joyful, 26–27
mozzarella cheese: Mediterranean
    Wraps with Garden
    Pesto, 169
Muffins, Bran, 152

ABOUT THE AUTHORS

Misty Copeland is a principal dancer at American Ballet Theatre. She is the author of the *New York Times* bestselling memoir *Life in Motion* and the award-winning children's book *Firebird*. Copeland made her Broadway debut in *On the Town*. She's been featured in the *New York Times*, on *60 Minutes*, and has been on the cover of *Essence* magazine. In 2014 she received a Dance Magazine Award, and was named one of *Self* magazine's Best Bodies. She was named, in 2015, one of *Time* magazine's 100 Most Influential People and a *Glamour* Woman of the Year.

Charisse Jones is a journalist and co-author of *Life in Motion*, *Unlocking the Truth: Three Brooklyn Teens on Life, Friendship and Making the Band*, and *Shifting: The Double Lives of Black Women in America*, winner of the American Book Award.

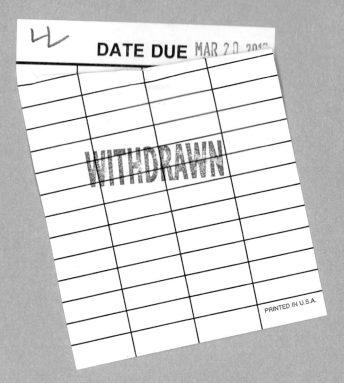